FEEDING
DEMONS

NICOLE GRANT

Feeding Demons

© 2014 by Nicole Grant

www.feedingdemonsbook.com

Cover art by Kim Voelker

Scripture quotations are from the New King James Version of the bible.

ISBN 978-0-9863613-3-3

www.ardeolit.com

ACKNOWLEDGMENTS

All the praise and glory for this work goes to God, first and foremost, as He made this possible. My hope is that I have been able to fulfill my responsibility as a good and faithful servant.

Thanks to my husband, whose support and encouragement always showed up at the exact moment I was in need, and for standing beside me during the most difficult of tribulations. And of course, for the chocolate tour.

Thanks to my early readers who each offered their own insights and motivation to help me both fine tune and trudge onward towards completion.

A big thank you to my cover artist, Kim Voelker, for capturing my vision and working hard to meet my specific demands. You have quite an artistic talent that truly amazes me.

Contents

INTRO

Food can be grouped into two categories, natural (God-made) and processed (man-made). God-made foods are those that are found abundantly in nature. Fruits, vegetables, grains, nuts, meats, fish, etc. are the foods that help keep our bodies functioning properly and at optimal health. Man-made foods are typically packaged in plastic. They are laden with chemicals and preservatives and contain high amounts of fat, sugar, and sodium; commonly and collectively they are known as junk food.

It has become widespread knowledge that America is an over-processed nation and many other countries are following suit. Fast food restaurants populate nearly every city and are more frequently popping up on street corners across the world. Our grocery stores are stocked full of pre-packaged junk foods made of chemicals we can't pronounce, let alone identify, while the fresh produce sections seem miniscule in comparison to the aisles upon aisles of detrimental chow.

Research is continually linking these man-made junk foods to our declining health. Obesity, diabetes, heart disease, and various types of cancers are some of the most common and most life-threatening health risks related to diet. Children are not exempt either. Childhood obesity, diabetes, heart disease, hypertension, and Attention Deficit Hyperactivity Disorder are all on the rise, yet can be alleviated through diet.

Ignorance is no longer an excuse. Gone are the days when we could blindly trust food production companies, grocery stores, and the government to safeguard our nutritional health and safety. National campaigns have been started to educate people on their food choices and the consequences of those decisions. We are bombarded with nutritional information constantly; on the television, internet, and billboards; in books, magazines, schools, stores, medical offices, hospitals, and often in the work place. Fast food restaurants are even capitalizing on the movement by offering their version of so-called healthy choices.

The information required to make proper nutritional decisions in order to improve your health and that of your loved ones is readily available at your fingertips. It mainly boils down to the common sense teachings that our ancestors have been handing down throughout the generations, which is to eat our fruits and veggies. Science has come a long way in terms of determining which particular foods hold more or less nutritional value, but basic knowledge remains the same. If it lives and grows on the earth, in most cases, we should consume it to help us survive and flourish.

You are probably already aware of what you should be eating, but for some reason you can't seem to stick to it. The big question is—why? Why do so many people opt for foods low in nutritional value which only succeed in harming their health? Why do we feed chemicals and unhealthy fats to ourselves, our families and friends, even our children? Is it simply taste? Do junk foods taste that much better, despite the fact that scientists spend countless hours in laboratories in an attempt to mimic flavors found in nature? Are we addicted to additives? Do our cravings stem from a perfectly achieved balance of high-fructose corn syrup and Red Dye #40? Is it really the ease of obtaining junk foods that are so readily available? Does it actually take longer to rinse off an apple than it does to open a bag of potato chips? Or is it something bigger? Is it something beyond our scope of everyday mortal life? Could there be an enemy so conniving as to turn one of our most basic necessities into a weapon of war to be used on ourselves, by ourselves? When we pull into that drive-thru or plunge into that bag of candy are we feeding and nourishing a hunger within our bodies, or are we simply feeding demons?

CHAPTER 1

THEY DON'T CALL IT DEVIL'S FOOD FOR NOTHING

"And the Lord God said to the woman, 'What is this you have done?'

The woman said, 'The serpent deceived me, and I ate,'" Genesis 3:13.

He has been using the tactic since the beginning of time and most of us are completely unaware. We blame ourselves, our genes, our careers, even our families, but have we ever turned our focus onto the real root of the problem? We have a tendency to point a finger at the nearest scapegoat and then refuse to look beyond the tip. How can we realistically expect to create a solution when we fail to see the origin of the crisis?

What if there was one reason people overeat? One reason people are overweight or obese? One reason people consistently find themselves reaching for cookies instead of carrots? Would we stop searching for health in a pill? Would we put an end to the years of yo-yo dieting, eating bland foods, and starving ourselves sick? Would we stop trying to find excuses and instead work on battling this one problem? There is someone to blame when it comes to the overindulgence of inadequate dietary choices and it's not your grocer or your

7

parent. You are battling an enemy who will use any means necessary to accomplish his goal. You are at war with an adversary for whom no tactic is too low, who has no moral compass, who will stop at nothing. He will use, abuse, manipulate, and deceive you until you are beaten, desperate, broken, and miserable. Who can be so malicious as to thrive on your pain and misery? Only the personification of evil himself.

Consideration has been given to the devil's use of drugs, alcohol, and pornography, but little attention has been paid to the fact that Satan has been using food against us since the dawn of human time. *"For the devil has sinned from the beginning,"* 1 John 3:8. He teases us, tempts us, and tortures us without our knowledge of what is going on. The devil and his minions have seemingly perfected the art of food war. They go to battle today armed, not with bullets and bombs, but with chocolates and pastries. Heart-stopping fats and organ polluting preservatives are prettily packaged as cherry pies and pepperoni pizzas, with most people being none the wiser to their toxic ingredients. To vividly see Lucifer in action, we can look back to the Garden of Eden. Satan used food in his first attack on mere mortals and ended up being immensely successful.

"Now the serpent was more cunning than any beast of the field which the Lord God had made. And he said to the woman, 'Has God indeed said, "You shall not eat of every tree of the garden?"'

And the woman said to the serpent, 'We may eat the fruit of the trees of the garden, but of the fruit of the tree which is in the midst of the garden, God has said, "You shall not eat it, nor shall you touch it, lest you die."'

Then the serpent said to the woman, 'You will not surely die,'" Genesis 3:1-4.

When we hear the story, we tend to take away the general lesson; Satan will try to tempt us, but we should not fall victim to his

9

trickery. We tend to view the fruit as symbolic of knowledge and power, but if we were to look at it in a more literal way, it's very simple to imagine ourselves in the very same scenario in modern day times. Perhaps Eve was simply hungry and looking for a snack. God had made it clear that one particular tree had some bad fruit with a nasty side effect (today's version might be a plate of nachos piled with the works and washed down with a frothy chocolate milkshake). Along comes the serpent to make it sound tasty ("Just look at that gooey cheese . . .") and like so many of us today, Eve fell for it. We know she didn't die right away, but we don't know if she was plagued by high cholesterol or struggled constantly to lose those stubborn extra ten pounds.

The story of Adam and Eve is routinely taught and interpreted in a complex and insightful manner. It is the moment at which the decline of human society began. It is the first time people blatantly disobeyed God. It is not a lighthearted story. It is not my intention to take anything away from the teachings of good and evil, nor am I suggesting the breadth of the story is not as wide as it has always been preached. Rather, I'm asking you to take a step back and take an additional look at it in a more simplified, straightforward, and literal way.

Eve is standing in a beautiful garden, staring at a tree that produces a food that is toxic to humans. The food is not healthy and it will cause ruinous side effects. The food is poisonous. It looks good, it smells good, but it will make her sick from the inside out. The food that this tree produces will damage her vital organs. It will corrupt her heart, brain, liver, kidneys, everything. The produce that she sees on this tree is going to make her miserable and snatch her life from her much sooner and in a more painful way than necessary. When Eve takes a bite of this fruit, she is knowingly taking one step towards death. She is willingly ingesting food that our Creator warned would lead to her demise. Why? Why would she take a bite? Why would she offer a taste to her loved one? She knows what this food will do to them. She has been warned *not* to eat this particular food by God Himself. She is surrounded by an abundance of healthy, viable options to satisfy her hunger. Why on earth would she choose to eat the one thing that will speed up her death and cause misery? *Because the snake told her she would be fine.* She was duped, lied to, tricked, deceived and she chose to believe the conniving snake over her heavenly Father. Now, before you start throwing stones and judging Eve as gullible, daft, disloyal, and the myriad of other not-so pleasantries running through your mind, take a long, hard look in the mirror. When you go to your local grocery store, *you* are Eve in the garden. When you load your shopping cart full of chips, cookies, frozen dinners, and pints of ice cream (even if there is a buy one get one free sale and the label says fat-free) you are sinking to the exact same level as Eve in Eden. We were supposed to learn a lesson from Eve's horrible mistake. The bible reiterates Satan's evil intent in John 8:44, *"He was a murderer from the beginning, and does not stand in the truth, because there is no truth in him. When he speaks a lie, he speaks from his own resources, for he is a liar and the father of it."* We should have ascertained how to spot the enemy's transparent deceit from a mile away, especially when he uses one of our basic necessities against us. Judging by the increasing amount of love handles and muffin tops however, it seems we have thus far failed to take away any understanding from Eve's saga.

Every grocery store is stocked with fruits, vegetables, and other foods that will make you healthier, happier, and quite possibly allow you to live longer, but it is also stocked full of nutritiously vacant junk that will harm your body. Are you choosing healthy, nourishing foods or are you listening to Satan's tired old line that surely you will be fine? You know those potato chips are bad for you. You know the cookies and crackers are making you fat and miserable. You know the candy and sodas are literally eating away at your insides. You know this. You have been warned repeatedly, by many different sources. Why do you choose foods that hurt you? Why do you pick foods that are killing you? Because Satan is telling *you* that you will be fine, you will not surely die. You are being duped, lied to, tricked, deceived, and *you* are choosing to believe it. When you consciously make the decision to stock up on boxed dinners full of preservatives and candy for dessert you are no better than Eve. You are deliberately ignoring your Creator's instructions to treat your body as a temple and fill it with wholesome, healthy foods. Granted, death may not be instantaneous, but every empty calorie and every chemical additive you ingest brings you one step closer to a painful demise and one step further from honoring your loving Father.

Grocery stores are not the only battlefield where the enemy launches his attacks. It's an all too familiar story for many of us today—we wander into our kitchens in search of a snack and out pops that pint of rocky road. We know we should snack on something more nutritious, but then we hear the enemy reminding us of how sweet that fudge swirl is. All too often, many of us give in to temptation and binge on food that has little or no health value. By now we are all aware of the physical damage we are inflicting upon our bodies with poor eating habits, and sadly, many people decide to live with it, albeit in a depressed or negative state of mind. You are miserable and God is grieving, while Satan is happily profiting from your malnutrition and physical deterioration.

There is an even greater danger beyond expanding waistlines, and it is Satan's ulterior motive for causing you physical pain and suffering. We must keep in mind that Satan's ultimate goal is to keep us from being close to God. He will use whatever he can to try and knock us off our paths—doubt, temptation, guilt, and fear to name a few of the obvious. He will not hesitate to utilize any method possible to achieve his goal of separating us from the Father. Using food to tempt seems to be the devil's weapon of choice. Culinary persuasion is a tried and true method the enemy has used to his advantage for centuries. It is so powerful that Satan even used it as his first attack on Jesus. *"Then Jesus was led up by the Spirit into the wilderness to be tempted by the devil. And when He had fasted forty days and forty nights, afterward He was hungry. Now when the tempter came to Him, he said, 'If you are the Son of God, command that these stones become bread,'"* Matthew 4:1-3.

Tempting Jesus would be no easy feat, so it makes sense for Satan to use his most powerful weapon first. Surprisingly, it's not riches, nor power, but plain old bread. Jesus, during His stay on earth, was a man and after forty days, He was hungry. If we skip lunch one afternoon, by six o'clock even cardboard starts to sound appetizing. You can well imagine that after more than a month without any edible sustenance, Christ was probably quite eager for a bite to eat. Satan wasted no time in pouncing on Jesus's empty stomach. He tried to get Christ to defy our Lord and Creator with a loaf of bread, way to bring out the big guns, right? He's up against the Son of man and the master of evil taunts Him with a nice freshly baked pillow of dough, warm and yeasty, surrounded by a golden flakey crust. How easy is it for you to walk into a bakery first thing in the morning and forgo the fluffy blueberry muffins, buttery croissants, and gooey banana bread? Walking out with *only* a four hundred calorie syrup-laden latte would be a feat in and of itself for most of us. He's Christ and He's perfect, so it goes without saying that He had enough stamina to resist a loaf of bread. Of course Christ was able to resist the temptation, but sadly, most of us do not even try.

Jesus fasted forty days and forty nights and still refused the urge to eat the devil's offerings. We go to a restaurant and stuff ourselves with a bountiful three course meal and yet we cannot find the will power to turn down dessert. Besides being sinless, Christ also had another huge edge that scripture points out, one that is vital and must not be ignored or overlooked; the Spirit had led Him to be tempted by the devil. Jesus knew what was coming. He was aware that Satan would try to tempt Him with food. Until now, you probably haven't realized that every time you open your refrigerator door you are facing the same attack Christ faced in the wilderness. Satan is sitting inside, waiting to turn your attention away from the vitamin-packed juice and towards the chemical-laden soda instead. It's hardly a fair fight when the assailant remains hidden and it's nearly impossible to win a war when you don't know who your opponent is. Now you know who is behind the attempted assaults and you can face the onslaughts head on. No longer do you need to blindly go into battle to face an unknown enemy. Bravely face your foe and his sinful offerings of cookies, pies, cakes, candy, chips, and any other junk food he throws your way and deny his ambush.

For far too many of us, Satan has been successful at launching his sneak attacks. The simple reason for his massive success is that we aren't even aware he is harassing us. In our society of excess, Satan and his henchmen have done a very good job of fattening us up, thereby clogging our arteries and making us miserable. Now that obesity has become an epidemic and we can no longer deny there is a problem affecting the majority of our citizens, he has astutely altered his strategy to keep those blinders firmly in place. He has managed to keep the heat off himself as the root cause of the problem. "Yes, we're fat, but it's not our fault!" is the new battle cry. Blame the fast food industry, blame a genetic defect, blame our parents, but let's not blame the Angel of darkness and our own gullibility in believing him.

There is hope, however, and evil can be defeated. Knowing the true enemy is a key component in waging a successful counter attack. You can now stop feeding the demons and begin to free yourself from Satan's clutches. Simply being aware of the culinary temptation you are facing puts you on a whole new playing field. You can face the devil and his evil antics utilizing the same power Christ used to help shield yourself from his contemptible aggressions, because with God all things are possible. However, you can no longer swim in the bliss of ignorance. You now know whom you are fighting and his weaponry of choice. You can choose to be rebellious like Eve in the garden and remain under Satan's spell or you can be Christ in the wilderness and tell the evil one to take a hike and reclaim your freedom from his grasp.

For another shining example of someone resisting the temptations of food we can look to Daniel's story in the Old Testament. *"But Daniel purposed in his heart that he would not defile himself with the portion of the king's delicacies, nor with the wine which he drank,"* Daniel 1:8. To summarize, Daniel was offered up some of the king's delicacies to partake in, and you can well imagine the king must have had quite the spread. There was probably an endless supply of scrumptious foods to choose from. However, Daniel knew that these foods had been offered to pagan idols, thus, they were tainted by evil. Understanding that the king's delicacies had direct ties to the devil drove Daniel to flat out refuse the food and fast for ten days, simply to earn the right to consume only vegetables and water. As a result of Daniel and his fellow servants' obedience to God, they were spiritually rewarded, for *"God gave them knowledge and skill in all literature and wisdom; and Daniel had understanding in all visions and dreams,"* Daniel 1:17.

We can easily use Daniel as a demonstration of not letting evil spirits use provisions to disempower and harm us. Daniel was aware of the true enemy behind the offering of the delicacies and he took a stand against Satan. Daniel relied upon God to keep him healthy during the fast and to orchestrate a way to have pure, clean sustenance free from sinful temptation. Similar situations apply to us today. How often do we attend parties catered with an endless supply of junk food? We are free to indulge ourselves with heaps and heaps of fodder and wash it down with a few beers or sodas from an abundantly stocked cooler. People are known to snack incessantly on the hors d'oeuvres simply because they are in front of them, readily available, provided by their kind and gracious host, much like the generous king was doing for Daniel. I imagine it bears a striking resemblance to many a soiree you have attended, doesn't it? Granted your host more than likely did not perform a pre-ceremony dedication of the chips and dip to pagan gods, but you must ask yourself who influenced the variety of available appetizers? Does the bounty appear as though it was supplied by Christ, meant to nourish and feed your bodily temple? Or does the selection seem offered by someone else, meant to afford you the chance to gluttonously stuff yourself with fats and sugars to the point of physical discomfort and regret?

Another noteworthy point in this particular story of Daniel and the others was that even after starving themselves for ten days, they visibly appeared more healthy and vibrant than those who had consumed the king's delicacies. We've all heard the old adage, you are what you eat, and this particular instance is a prime example. Those who divulged in the sin-tainted delicacies paid for it in their appearance and vigor. We live in a highly vain society, where too much emphasis is placed on looks, however the scripture is not referring to Daniel and his cohorts as simply being tanned and toned, ready to model for the hottest fitness magazines. There is a deeper meaning that goes beyond the surface and should not be glazed over lightly. The men looked healthier on the exterior because they were healthier on the interior. What we put into our bodies shows up on the outside. Daniel and his men did not poison their bodies with the pagan-dedicated food and as a result, they were superior to those that did eat the junk food on both a physical and spiritual level, from the inside out. Staying away from food that has been tainted by the devil in any way, shape or form can only have positive results on multiple levels.

I hope things are beginning to click into place for you, that you are now beginning to see your food and weight issue in a new light. I pray that you would remove the scales from your eyes to clearly see your enemy for the snake he is and take up arms to fend off his vicious attacks on your physical and spiritual well-being. Unfortunately, spiritual warfare can be easy to ignore because we simply cannot *see* it in front of our face and typically there is no tangible evidence until we are severely beaten. I assure you, it is there and the proof is becoming quite obvious thanks to ever-increasing pant sizes. Every gastronomic temptation placed before you is a strategically planned attack on you personally, for your very soul. Every time you cave and pop that wicked morsel into your mouth you are increasing Satan's arsenal against you and strengthening the evil one's control over you, creating separation from your Father and shuffling you towards physical death. Now I ask, are you ready to recapture culinary control and stop feeding demons?

CHAPTER 2
HELL'S IN YOUR KITCHEN

"Be sober, be vigilant; because your adversary the devil walks about like a roaring lion, seeking whom he may devour," 1 Peter 5:8.

We have been forewarned, the devil is out to get us; each and every one of us. No one is excluded, he'll take whoever he can get. Many of us choose to ignore this warning and pretend we're perfectly safe in our pleasant little lives. We delude ourselves into believing that evil cannot or will not touch us. Of course we know evil exists, one merely has to turn on the news to witness the atrocious happenings of daily life. For the purpose of this book, I'm not referring to the grand-scale evil acts that shock and appall. I want to address the subtle, sneaky acts of malevolence committed against us on a regular, daily basis. We diet and remain fat. We exercise yet the numbers on the scale don't change. We have ourselves sliced open to vacuum out the fat or clamp our stomach and still the weight remains. Excess fat is not the enemy, it is merely the bullet that causes the damage. If fat is the bullet—who's holding the gun?

One of the scariest things about the enemy

is that he doesn't seem to need a lot of immediate fanfare. For someone who pushes instant gratification, he certainly has a handle on his patience and perseverance. Surprisingly, he does not even appear to have a narcissistic obsession with getting credit for all the evil committed in this world. This makes him all the more dangerous because he is content to quietly, slowly, and shrewdly inflict damage. Destruction through your diet is one such example, as the effects of poor dietary choices are rarely seen right away. It can take years before the results of eating junk food become apparent, sometimes not becoming visible for entire decades.

Satan wants you fat. Why? Every moment you spend thinking about your body, your weight, food you should eat, food you shouldn't eat, is a moment taken away from thoughts of God. God gave you life for a purpose and it wasn't to count calories. How many hours, days, weeks, even years of your life have been dedicated to dieting, to losing weight, and all the struggles that go with it? Isn't there something more positive and productive you could have done with that time? The devil cares about your weight because the heavier you are, the less healthy you are and the easier it is for him to influence you, corrupt you, and keep you from your purpose. Don't let what you weigh get in your way. Rarely do you find someone who is overweight, truly happy, and leading a full life. The only example I can think of is Jolly old St. Nick. Yes, he's plump and happy and gives presents to all the girls and boys. The legend of Santa perpetuated a myth that fat people are supposed to be jolly, but in truth that's about as believable as a man who delivers toys to the entire world in one night.

Why does Satan want us miserable? Because God urges us to be joyful. Satan wants what God doesn't. It's black and white, good and evil, there are no shades of gray. Satan is unequivocally the polar opposite of God. If the Lord wants to see us joyful, healthy, happy, and loving, it stands to reason that the devil wants to see us miserable, suffering, hurting, and in pain. The enemy delights in our demise, the more wretched we are, the happier he is. His biggest, most crucial intention is to keep us from our Lord. What the devil wants most is to see us apart from our Creator. It's easy to fall into the trap of believing the devil won't bother us. His work is transparent in the neighbor's house, where their teen stays out partying all night, addicted to drugs and it's even plain to see the devil influencing the alcoholic three cubicles over. Yes, Satan does make some of his work prominent in our society, but let's not forget how subtle he can be at times. He wants a piece of you, my friend, and if a pastry is the way to get it, how sweet is that?

Many believers of Christ are easily lulled into a false sense of safety because we know we are spoken for, bought and paid for. We've announced Jesus as our Lord and Savior, so we're safe, right? The devil can't touch us. I'm sure Job would have something different to say about that. Being a Christian does not render us untouchable; we are still highly susceptible to attacks by the evil one. Satan is incessantly trying to knock us off our spiritual paths, doing whatever he can to try and separate us from the Lord. It is our job to be aware, be watchful, and constantly be on the lookout for his ruses. We must be alert, waiting for him to pounce, and, given the increasing extra poundage in our society, too many of us are failing miserably.

When most people are overweight and fighting with their diets, it certainly seems they do not turn towards God. They will look to a pill, a book, a speedy new exercise, a surgical procedure, or a magical shake, but they don't seem to be laying their weight issues at the feet of Christ. Maybe they believe it's not

33

significant enough, maybe they're stubbornly trying to handle it themselves, or maybe they're too ashamed. Whatever the reason, it's erroneous. Many people, when faced with huge disasters, traumas or difficulties in their lives will turn to God in a heartbeat. By slowly torturing us, Satan tries to push us to the edge of our limits, to make us as miserable as humanly possible, before we decide to turn to God. Once we unburden ourselves and relinquish the issue to the Lord, the devil has lost, and this is obviously not what the enemy wants. The devil is remarkably patient and content to work slowly, relying on the fact that over time, people become more and more complacent. It has taken decades for the US to become the fattest nation. Not so very long ago, larger people were in the minority and they suffered ridicule, harsh judgment, and discrimination. Unfortunately, these injustices still happen, however, being overweight has become the norm and we are often encouraged to merely accept the extra weight individuals carry around. While no one deserves to be mocked or insulted for their size, by not speaking out and trying to help them, we are simply ignoring the problem and inflicting hurt through our silence. Obviously fat is not a laughing matter. It's not something to insult people for, but it is an issue we need to assist people with. Oftentimes simply talking with someone and addressing their unhealthy lifestyle is a difficult, yet important first step. Avoiding obesity does not make it disappear. Ignoring the extra pounds, and all of the accompanying health issues, will not make them start to suddenly melt away.

One of, if not the major theme of this book, is the importance of awareness. We must be conscious of excess weight and how unhealthy it is. We must be aware of the devil's desire to get you fat and keep you there. Once you acknowledge the enemy is attacking you with foods it becomes glaringly obvious how and when he strikes against you. In those moments, once you begin to realize an attempt is being made to torture you with treats, you will quickly wise up and thus be more successful in withstanding the temptation.

It's really no wonder that so many people feel they're losing their battles with weight loss. The battle is not against food and it's not against your own self, but rather versus the Angel of Darkness. The instigator of iniquity has you targeted in his sights. You are battling the devil and his demons, and that is why it's so hard. That is why you "fail" over and over again. Your enemy is the epitome of evil and you don't even know you're being attacked! Do you see why it has been next to impossible to stay consistent with changing your eating habits? Satan is definitely a skilled opponent, especially when he's leading super-secret spy operations against you. The good news is that you now know who it is that you're up against; now it's time you start to be on the lookout for his attacks and become hyper-vigilant about when he wages war against you. Do you know where Satan lurks, waiting for you? Are you conscious of the culinary attacks he's launching on you? Let's take a look at some common places the demons may be waiting to strike.

Remember playing hide-and-seek as a child and learning that sometimes the most obvious hiding place is also the best? Satan figured that trick out a long time ago. Food is never hard to find in our daily lives, we eat it three or more times a day. We need food to fuel our bodies. What better place to launch an attack on you both physically and spiritually than via something you're exposed to every day, multiple times a day? Who would expect the food you buy at your local supermarket to be a weapon of destruction? Who would anticipate demons to be lurking in the fluffy depths of a pretty pink frosted cupcake? No one. We do not equate food with evil in modern society, yet it can and does inflict a tremendous amount of harm upon us when not properly consumed, and that is why Satan has chosen to use it to destroy you.

Our home is supposed to be our haven. It's where we go for peace, comfort, and rest. I hate to break it to you, but your safe house has been breached. How do I know? Look in your cupboards. Are they full of packaged foods? Chips, cookies, cereals, candy? Look a little further; what's on the ingredient list? Can you pronounce everything you put into your body? Now how does your produce stash compare? Don't think for a second that it counts if you buy a ton of fresh produce only to end up feeding it to the garbage disposal because it went rotten before you ate it. Satan is actively engaging in warfare in your very own home. Does the devil really hang out in your cupboards? Yes. If you have a weakness for food, he will most certainly take up lodging between the licorice and chips. Whenever you go into your own kitchen for a snack, you are entering the devil's playground. It sounds so dramatic, but take a look down—is your belly protruding? Belt buckled into the last possible hole? Are elastic waistbands leaving imprints on your skin? Those are the visible side effects of allowing Satan to take up residence in your pantry.

The enemy attacks a lot of people when they sit down to watch television. Your hands are idle, your brain has happily zoned off, and the devil has a nice noisy box, complete with flashing lights to garner your attention and send you subliminal messages to eat unhealthy snacks. For many people it has become an ingrained habit to mindlessly chow down while watching TV. It's quite common to sit in front of the screen, noshing on your potato chips, when suddenly an ice cream commercial appears and sends you digging through the frosty depths of your freezer in search of some gooey swirling fudge-laced bliss. The next commercial break teases you with candy and suddenly you're off in search of your chocolate bar stash. What will the next hour hold? Soda? Beer? Excessively buttered microwave popcorn? The abundance of products marketed is endless.

What about mealtimes? Does the devil frequently convince you that it's easier and quicker to gobble down takeout or pre-packaged meals? Do you often find yourself falling prey to this fallacy because you're tired and stressed out? Who wants to go home and lovingly prepare a feast full of fresh ingredients that will only nourish you and your body when you can just stop for some previously frozen, sodium-laden, heart stopping grub handed to you in a greasy paper bag? Sure, the enemy paints a pretty picture of ease and convenience, but at what cost? Ironically, most of the quick and easy foods we devour due to lack of time and effort will actually deplete our energy level and leave us feeling more tired and stressed.

Do you think the devil might like to hang out around your place of work to tantalize you with treats? How often do well-meaning co-workers bring in donuts, cookies, candy, cake, etc. to share? Are there vending machines stocked full of sodas and plastic wrapped goodies? What about company parties? Are they catered with fresh fruits and veggies, or pizza, chips, and pre-made sodium sandwiches on bleached white bread? Do you see the devil's handiwork loitering on your commute to and from work? Food billboards litter America's roadways, while large-scale signs decorate the sides of trains, buses, and even buildings themselves. Radio commercials you hear on your drive propagate food temptations and incentives. It's a pretty safe assumption that Satan and his demons don't mind accompanying you on your nine to five.

What about when you watch your favorite sports team? Typical stadium fare is laden with greasy calories that are harder on your heart than a home team defeat. Let's not forget the outrageously over-priced beer and soda we commonly purchase to wash down our indulgences. Prefer to watch the game from the comfort of your own couch? Try counting the number of alcohol and food advertisements during the next game and I'm sure you'll be astounded. There is, of course always the option of watching sports games at the local bars and pubs—you'd never expect to find the devil in one of those upstanding establishments, right?

Here's another scary place Satan manages to sneak into on a tray of sugary cookies: church gatherings. Well-meaning people provide refreshments before and after church services that have little to no nutritional value. Small group gatherings all too often revolve around unhealthy dinners or desserts and very easily overshadow the real intention of the assembly. I personally have seen too many churches putting out cakes, cookies, donuts, sodas, pastries, and brownies all in the name of love. I'm not questioning the motivation, I'm shedding light on the fact that these well-meaning provisions are more than likely not God given if they are unhealthy and cause more bodily harm than good. If a large percentage of the congregation is facing a weight issue, you can be sure Satan has gotten a foothold on the refreshment table. If you're the well-meaning bearer of baked goodies, what does that mean? Are you subconsciously an evil cohort? No, of course not. Everyone knows that when you donate a plate of brownies for the church bake sale you only have the best of intentions at heart. What you do need to know is that the devil is using you as a delivery service. He's sneaky, he's cunning, and he's tricking you into believing you're doing God's work by bringing in a box of sugar bombs that have the potential to destroy. Don't feel guilty, conflicted, or confused. Know the possible damage these unhealthy treats can inflict upon others and stand up to the enemy's suggestion that you bring a box of donuts in. Fight the devil by bringing in fruits, veggies, or at least fresh treats that have been baked from scratch, ideally with some healthful benefits. You will encounter resistance, you will have to listen to naysayers, and people will ignore your efforts. Pay no attention, they are engulfed in their own war and probably aren't aware of Satan's culinary grasp on them.

Another popular hangout for the devil is, of course, any type of party atmosphere. Family gatherings, friendly get-togethers, holiday celebrations, you name the occasion and he'll be there. Parties typically involve food and usually it's highly unhealthy food. Combine that with the fact that people tend to not pay attention to the amount of food they're consuming and it's a recipe for disaster. Many people will use festivities as an excuse to indulge. Sure, little Susie is turning five, but is it really necessary to have a heaping of ice cream nestled against your giant slice of cake as a chaser to the pizza, potato chips, and soda you had for dinner? Nope, that's just Satan egging you on to chow down all in the name of having a good time.

Where else is a regular haunt for the enemy? Restaurants of course! Fast food, family style, pubs, buffets; Satan has no preference, he'll frequent them all. Deceptively mouthwatering pictures adorn menus and even the walls of the building itself, but how often is what is served on your plate an actual replica of what was pictured? Rarely, if ever. Servings are typically enormously sized, prodding gluttony. The food itself is generally laden with salt and preservatives, as well as other unhealthy and questionable ingredients. When you do go to a restaurant try your best to find one geared towards serving healthy, fresh foods, or at the very least make some modifications to your order to increase the nutritional benefits. No matter what restaurant you decide to patron, you must enter with your full armor on. Be prepared to battle temptation and deception at some of the devil's finest.

You must become sober and vigilant. You must seriously figure out where you are most susceptible to assaults via your arteries. You need to identify where your enemy is lurking and you must anticipate his attacks. You must know that he is using food against you, keeping you unhealthy and creating a road-block in your spiritual life, which keeps you that much farther from experiencing true joy. The war for your spirit and your health is on, and your adversary is lurking in every cup-board, on every table, in every fridge, just waiting to tempt you.

CHAPTER 3
SATAN'S FOOD CHAIN

"Blessed is the man who endures tempta-tion; for when he has been approved, he will receive the crown of life which the Lord has promised to those who love Him. Let no one say when he is tempted, 'I am tempted by God,' for God can not be tempted by evil, nor does He Himself tempt anyone. But each one is tempted when he is drawn away by his own desires and enticed. Then, when desire has conceived, it gives birth to sin; and sin, when it is fully grown, brings forth death," James 1:12.

We are all tempted by food on a regular basis, although each of us possesses a unique palate. One person will crave the salty crunch of potato chips, another may savor the sweet bitterness of chocolate, and yet a third person will tell you they relish the warm, moist fluffiness of bread. There are as many diverse cravings as there are types of food. Although the items we are tempted by will vary drastically from person to person, the cycle each of us goes through remains fairly consistent. Satan's food chain is a cycle of thoughts, feelings, and events that can lead to personal destruction and, ultimately spiritual and physical death, as the bible blatantly tells us. God does not mince words, when we give into our own desires we are walking towards our own destruction. We're not talking about a peaceful, dying from old age type of death either, but years of unnecessary physical and mental anguish, surgeries, medications, hospital stays, endless torture and suffering that more and more people are accepting as a natural part of life. Is it possible to break this sequence and live a much less miserable, more highly satisfying life? Of course. First, however, we must be aware of the chain we get trapped in. You cannot break the cycle without consciously knowing about it and fighting to stay out. A quick overview of the different segments in Satan's food chain looks like this:

Temptation → Obsession → Desperation → Gluttony → Guilt → Denial → Pain and Death

Let's explore the different stages a little deeper so you can understand how he has been getting the best of you time and time again.

Temptation

Temptation is Satan's cheap shot. It's quick, easy, and works on most people the majority of the time. He figures out what we like and where we're weak and he attacks at the easiest point. The qualities of our favorite food become heightened. Chocolate is no longer dark, milk, or white; rather, it becomes a creamy, silky, smooth confection that melts in our mouth, bringing us to near ecstasy. Satan knows no boundaries of time or location either. For some of us he beckons from the office vending machine late in the afternoon. For others, he strikes late in the evening while we're watching television. Wherever, whenever, and whatever he's tempting you with, it's never easy to say no. Not only does he make the treat seem too tantalizing to refuse, he'll also fill your head with justifications, excuses, and bold-faced lies. Let's take a look at some of his more popular fabrications:

"I deserve it."

How many times have you resigned yourself to stick to a new diet and found success all week, only to have Friday roll around and you find yourself bombarded with options for guilty edible pleasures? You go out for a drink with coworkers and the frosty calories are sloshing in front of your face, or you're at home when you feel your defenses crumble as your spouse pulls out a bag of potato chips. Undoubtedly these treats are not a part of your healthy eating plan, yet you find yourself wrestling with temptation. It doesn't take long for you to decide that after a week of carrot sticks and salads, you're entitled to a reward. Unfortunately, you're not alone in your reasoning. The devil is able to convince us that being dedicated to good nutrition and health is not positive enough, we somehow "deserve" to sabotage our bodies by ingesting something completely void of nutritional value. Sadly, many of us are deceived and believe the lie that we are entitled to junk food over and over again. You must become aware of what the enemy is coercing you to believe. You are swallowing his lies that you deserve a large triple chocolate shake with your meal. He is blatantly duping you into believing that you're owed an extra-large fry because you worked overtime today. You ate healthy all week and now he wants you to believe that you deserve a double burger smothered with cheese and bacon.

Here's some cold, hard truth for you—you don't deserve it. You don't deserve to go to the drive thru for the third time this week. You don't deserve to add a side of onion rings. You don't deserve to have a second helping of red velvet cake. You don't deserve to snack on soda and chips. You don't deserve to eat the box of cookies. Put down the giant burrito loaded with cheese and sour cream because you DO NOT deserve it. Have I made my point?

Why do I say you are not fit for consuming whatever junk it is you crave? Change your backwards thinking right now—it is the garbage fodder that is not worthy of you. You do NOT deserve to eat these foods laden with fat, chemicals, sugars, sodium, artificial ingredients, etc., because you are a human being, made in the image of God. You are a person with thoughts, feelings, emotions, concerns, wants, dreams, hopes, and desires. *You deserve so much more.* You ought to have the highest quality of life, to enjoy life to the fullest and overeating non-nutritional foods is not the way to go about obtaining that.

When Satan convinces you to believe that you deserve a "treat," the reality behind that is actually one of misery and torture. Do you deserve to be on medication for high cholesterol? Do you warrant achy joints from your body's inability to eliminate years' worth of gastronomic overindulgence? Do you deserve a heart attack because there is too much fat built up around your internal organs? Is a needle every day justifiable because your body can no longer regulate insulin levels? Are you worthy of only feeling bloated, sluggish, depressed, and miserable? Posing the questions in a more truthful light makes the answers a no-brainer, right? The devil is asking you these very questions, only in a much more appealing way with a sweet, savory spin on it.

Ask yourself what you truly deserve and be brutally honest. Do you deserve to eat meals sure to induce heart disease and desserts laced with diabetes? No. Do you deserve to enjoy what you eat? Yes, absolutely—in a way that is beneficial to your body. We are talking about your quality of life. Realize that you are worthy of the best and be aware that you have an enemy who disagrees and will try anything to deceive you into believing otherwise.

<u>"Just a little bit won't hurt."</u>

Small amounts here and there won't do much damage and they allow us the opportunity to enjoy the culinary world. The problem arises when we fall for this line over and over again. A little bit of French fries on the side of a "small" greasy cheeseburger, followed by a gulp of milkshake does not equal a very nourishing meal, especially when you "only" had a chocolate chip muffin and three cups of coffee for breakfast. We have to be aware of how our "little bits" are adding up and we have to be conscious of how we define these "little bits." For one person, a small amount of ice cream is equivalent to half a cup, for someone else it might be half the carton. Guess who has a better perception of portion size? How do you know if you have a handle on your "little bits" or if you've simply fallen for Satan's lies too many times? The obvious answer is to look at your own physique. If you're not within an ideal weight range, then you're being led astray. If your health is not in good standing than you're being outright swindled.

One place to be really vigilant about portion control is at parties and large gatherings. The devil gets to kick back, relax, and enjoy the party. We end up distracting ourselves through conversation, and since most gatherings (good ones, anyway!) offer a generous selection of edibles, we easily lose track of just how much we've been eating. By the time you finish that conversation with Cousin Johnny, you've eaten your way through potato salad, pretzels, veggies and dip, trail mix, and Aunt Edna's homemade cheesecake bites and the main course hasn't even been served yet.

Want to know another place the devil lurks with this "little bit" lie? Ever been to a buffet style dinner? Yikes! You load different items on your plate a spoonful at a time and yet it's filled up before you're halfway through the line. Somehow, despite the fact that you've only gotten small amounts of each item, you end up with a heaping plate full of more food than you could possibly need in one day, let alone one meal.

The truth is, Satan will use this fib that a little bit won't hurt you anytime, anyplace and it's easy for him to get away with it. When we eat small amounts of junk food on occasion, it isn't overly harmful. The problem lies in the repetition and far too many of us are stuck on repeat. You need to know that when the false idea that just a little won't hurt rings in your head, it's not a blessing, it's not permission, it is a deliberate attack on your health meant to bring you harm, piece by piece.

"No one will ever know."

You've started a weight loss challenge with your family and friends so you can hold each other accountable. While out running errands, your favorite fast food restaurant beckons you toward its quick and discreet drive-thru. You know you shouldn't partake and you think of all the heckling you would get from your competition, but how would they ever find out? For some people, the only thing coming between them and a box of fudge is what others may think.

It's easy to find private moments throughout the day to cheat and stuff your face with your guilty pleasure of choice and, lest you forget, the devil has no qualms about reminding you. You can snag a cookie on the way to your office, and then double-back later for seconds when no one is around. You can stop at the store, pick up a bag of chips and soda, devour it in the car, and dispose of the remains without anyone being privy to your secret rendezvous. How many parents wait until their kids are at school to pilfer the candy bowl? When you're sneaking treats without anyone knowing they taste good for about thirty seconds while the flavors— mostly engineered in a lab, mind you—do a dance on your taste buds. Not a minute after you swallow the last bite you feel awful and ashamed. It is so indicative of human nature it's even mentioned in Proverbs 20:17, *"Bread gained by deceit is sweet to a man, but afterward his mouth will be filled with gravel."* The fact is, you know what you're shoving into your mouth and you are the one that has to live with yourself. You need to stop believing his little lie that "no one will know, so it won't hurt." It's hurting you! The greasy chicken legs you grabbed on the way home from work aren't clogging your spouse's arteries, they're clogging yours.

There are several truths that discount Satan's fib that no one will know. First, as mentioned earlier, *you* know how unhealthy your eating habits are. You are well aware when you overeat or when you're eating junk food that only brings harm to your body. It's easy to overlook this truth, to excuse it away, ignore it, or simply play dumb. However, it's obviously not doing you any good and it is past time you stop lying to yourself.

The second truth is that others do know and even suffer because of it. If you're obese, you can eat all the salads you want in front of people, they still know you eat a lot more than lettuce behind closed doors. Fat does not magically accumulate on your body. We all know it comes from overeating and consuming the nutritional equivalent of garbage or, in some instances, a medical condition that most likely can be alleviated through proper diet. Skipping dessert when you're dining out with friends is a noteworthy gesture, but if it simply leads you to the cookie jar when you get home, it's pointless. You are much better off sharing a dessert with your companion. Eating in secrecy in hopes that no one will know isn't working; you're not fooling anyone and the sooner you come to terms, the sooner you can release the devil's grip on your fork.

You may wonder how others suffer from your overeating. It is very difficult to watch someone you love inflict bodily harm upon themselves. It's not easy to observe someone you care about pile on the pounds and create an exhaustive list of medical and emotional problems, and it's not fun for others to see you in pain or despair. It's no simple task to look at someone subtracting years from their life and know that they're also shortchanging themselves in their quality of life as well. What if you're a parent? A grandparent? If you're unable to actively engage with them, do you realize you're robbing children of cherished memories? The truth is that others do know and they are affected, probably much more so than you realize. Don't be afraid to use the concern of others to help motivate you. Relish in the fact that improving your health has a ripple effect on those around you in countless ways.

The third truth is that God knows. You can go into the deepest, darkest closet, but He is still with you and He knows you're hurting yourself. Do you realize that when you're wounding yourself, you are hurting Him as well? We are God's children, His creation, and He does not want to see us suffer, yet we continually subject ourselves to treat-induced torture. You can't lie to God, you can't trick God, and you can't outwit Him. The good news is that He would love to help you end your misery. Never being alone means just that—you're never alone. God is there with you to provide a source of strength, should you ask, not to admonish you for delving into another bag of cheese puffs. God is the most important weapon in your arsenal, which we'll discuss later on. Just remember that no matter how lonely you feel you are not by yourself in this battle and know that Jesus can fully empathize with what you are going through. *"For in that He Himself has suffered, being tempted, He is able to aid those who are tempted,"* Hebrews 2:18.

"It doesn't matter."

Perhaps you've been on a diet but haven't seen any results so you start to believe eating an extra candy bar won't make things any worse. Maybe you think you're so overweight that one more bowl of ice cream isn't going to make a difference. Hopefully you're not under the impression that no one cares how unhealthy you are so a few more pounds won't change anything. If you regularly find yourself believing that it doesn't matter what you eat or how much you consume, you are a prime target for the enemy's attacks. Unfortunately, the devil is bombarding you and you're allowing him to beat you up both mentally and physically. There may be a completely unrelated issue you're dealing with in life that you believe is leading you to food, in which case he's simply kicking you while you're down. Whatever the case may be, it is critical that you realize right now that it does matter. It matters to you, otherwise you would not be reading this book and it matters to God, whose opinion you don't want to take lightly.

Probably one of the most common, yet harmful statements when it comes to changing eating patterns is, "I'll start tomorrow." The temptation to delay healthful eating stems from the lie that it doesn't matter. Perhaps it's lunch time and you're debating between a zesty Greek salad and a fattening gyro. Thinking of the donut you had for breakfast, you decide the day has already been thwarted and it won't matter if you just go with the artery-clogger today and try to improve your diet tomorrow. What's a few (hundred) more greasy calories? Familiar story? Why do I say it's so detrimental? First of all, as you probably know, that particular brand of "tomorrow" never comes for the vast majority of people. Think of how many times you've vowed to alter your eating habits the next day, or the following week, or January first. Do you believe you're the only one to make those appointments for your health and fail to show up? Typically people get distracted, busy, or simply lose motivation to make the culinary switch they promised themselves. All too often, tomorrow comes and goes, yet we've done nothing to make an improvement.

The second reason delaying is dangerous is the simple fact that you're on the clock. We all come with an expiration date and not knowing when that day is should put more pressure on you to start enjoying your life and living it to the fullest. Starting now gets you one day closer to better health, and better health may equate to more days for you here on earth. The only thing that doesn't matter is what you ate at your last meal. What does matter is that you stop listening to the lies and deceit and make a change now, today, for the better.

"Food is my comfort."

Of all the underhanded reasons to tempt you with food, comfort is perhaps the most dangerous. Thanks to the enemy's invisible influence on multiple daytime talk shows, millions of overeaters are now attributing their culinary desires to comfort. Eating because you are sad, lonely, mad, stressed, depressed, happy, or any other feeling on the emotional spectrum goes beyond the peril of merely having an excuse to gorge. The tip of the iceberg is to point out that eating for comfort is an unhealthy explanation you give yourself for picking up that fork, but the problem is much more serious than that. An excuse quickly becomes a reason and a reason turns into justification. If you find a way to justify your poor eating habits, you are in very grave danger. Once you can justify something, as harmful as it may be, it becomes harder for you to see reality and face the truth about your poor choices. If you find yourself making justifications or excuses about your unhealthy nutrition you need to do serious damage control on your thought process. Quit listening to the devil and start thinking for yourself.

On any given day, you might come home from a bad day at work only to end up in an argument with your spouse. Tired and frustrated, you pull out your trusty comrades who will never scale back your pay or leave dirty underwear on the floor, good old peanut butter and chocolate. There is undoubtedly a moment of hesitation before you pull off the wrapper when the thought crosses your mind that you shouldn't be doing this, knowing full well it's not going to solve your problems. Do you listen? Or do you simply dive in, reassuring yourself that it's your "comfort" and will make you feel better, at least for the time being? Obviously far too many of us are falling for the latter. Somewhere along the line, terms like "comfort food," "eating for comfort," and "food is my friend" turned from popular catch phrases into unhealthy validations. In truth, these excuses are simply a distraction. The enemy is distracting you with cozy, cuddly thoughts of sugars and sweets so you don't have to pay attention to what he's really doing.

The bible tells us we are to find solace and comfort in our Creator. When you are sad, lonely, depressed, or worried, God wants you to turn to Him. He is to be your ear to listen to your concerns, your shoulder to cry on and lean on; He is your confidant, your counselor, your friend, your Father. Listening to the devil tell you to eat a bowl full of nacho chips does not make things better. You may relish in five minutes of taste bud bliss, but what happens when the bag runs out? The answer to your original problem is not magically revealed; your concerns and worries have not miraculously disappeared. You are worse off than when you started nibbling away because now you're feeling bloated and gaseous in addition. Sounds really consoling, right?

When Satan is enticing you to seek solace in food rather than your Father, he is leading you to outright disobedience. It's easy to see defiance when we think of unhealthy eating in terms of gluttony and relinquishing into temptation, but when you're in pain and turn to a pie it's also a form of waywardness that's just a little harder to realize. You must be aware of the enemy's shrewdness. He will gladly befriend you in the form of oily French fries to lead you astray.

Obsession

Once Satan has successfully tempted us

with an unhealthy food or beverage, it begins to invade our mind and we wind up obsessing. For some, those who lose their battle quickly, the obsession stage does not last very long, while others will endure for days on end before giving in. You know you are obsessing when nothing else seems to satisfy your hunger, if you can't seem to think of anything else, or if you find yourself waking in a cold sweat in the middle of the night yearning to head towards the kitchen.

How often do you get a taste for a double cheeseburger, but opt not to have it because you know it's not what you need, when suddenly you're driving home from work and every other billboard you see is an advertisement for a burger joint? Restaurant signs seem to glow a bit brighter than all the other lights and even the radio is singing jingles to encourage you to stop and grab a slab of beef on a bun. Yes, once we start obsessing over some form of food, messages seem to pop up left and right, pointing us in the exact direction we don't want to go. Some may say this is purely coincidence, others will argue that you're just paying more attention to those particular signs, but I say it is the enemy hard at work. At times, especially in the beginning, it's difficult to make the healthy choice. Satan and his minions are right there, desperately trying to throw you off track and keep your mind on junk food. They'll flash you pretty pictures or find ways to whisper sweet nothings, anything to convince you that you need to fill your belly with garbage.

Typically, our first line of defense while in the obsessive stage is to eat everything else we can possibly think of. Fortunately, a lot of people will make an effort to choose healthier options than whatever the item of desire is. Unfortunately, stuffing ourselves full of miscellaneous foods only to end up binging on the obsessed-over item anyway is extremely counterproductive. All too often, that is precisely what ends up happening. It's late in the evening, you're watching television and you keep thinking about that bag of salty potato chips sitting in the cupboard. Determined not to eat them, you browse through the fridge and find an apple instead. Five minutes after you polish off the apple, your mind is still on those chips. Still unwavering, you go back and grab a bag of peanuts; they're salted, so they should put an end to the chip craving, right? Nope, ten minutes later you still have chips on the brain. Now what? Perusing the pantry, trying to avoid even looking at the offenders, you spot some multigrain crackers. They're kind of chip-like but offer a bit of nutrition so you grab some of those. You know how this story line ends, despite any attempts at healthier snacks you still end up digging into the bag of greasy fried potato slices. You see, when the enemy wants you to obsess over something he is quite adept at being relentlessly persistent.

Rely on your skills of ignoring and avoiding. If you need to, tell him out loud to leave you alone. Sure, your sanity may come into question, but do whatever it takes to chase the demons away.

Some people will attempt distraction with other activities like doing a workout, cleaning the house, reading a book, anything to get their mind off of food. When these tactics work, it is inarguably a huge plus. If you can find a healthy interest to distract you, that is fabulous and something you should hold on to, as long as you don't end up fixating on the activity itself. Replacing one obsession with another is quite counterproductive.

Satan loves when we obsess because if our mind is on food, it is not on God. The enemy enjoys seeing us dejected, he takes great pleasure in seeing us suffer, but most of all, he loves seeing us apart from our Creator. Remind yourself of this next time you can't seem to get your mind off of a large tub of movie style popcorn. Kudos if you obsess over a pint of ice cream and manage to not overindulge in it, but don't lose sight of the fact that even if you're successful in your junk food avoidance, by spending precious time and energy analyzing it, you have at least partly played into the devil's hands anyway. Learn to recognize obsession for what it is. It's not a nutritional deficiency, nor just a sweet tooth. It is Satan's way of keeping you distracted, guiding your thoughts and emotions to keep your mind off track of where it should be. Cease the enemy before he turns your simple thoughts into obsessions and you'll feel more satisfied for it. Not only will you feel sated, you'll avoid falling into the next step of Satan's food chain.

Desperation

The devil never fails to get a chuckle at us while we are desperate. The constant obsessing eventually causes us to crack and the results can range from moderate to severe. Desperation may lead us to do something as trivial as "borrowing" a candy bar from our kids' stash, something as disgusting and utterly humiliating as digging through the garbage to make sure that empty bag of pretzels was really empty, or it can lead to a middle of the night shopping trip. Ever wonder why it's necessary for drive-thru's to be open until 2 a.m.? Uncontrollable late night cravings don't seem to be just for pregnant ladies anymore.

When we can no longer fight the urge, we become desperate. Whether you've spent days, hours, or mere minutes struggling to resist the temptation, once you succumb to it, your mind is no longer simply invaded, but it is under control. The world around you ceases to exist as you make your way to the kitchen, preparing to dive into a bag of gummy bears and unable to stop yourself. Your work out buddy can't help you, your spouse can't come to your aid, there is no one to stop you from caving and giving in to your sinful desire. Desperation kicks in the moment you decide to relinquish control and feed the demons. It happens the second you opt to listen to the devil. He gets excited and he takes the reins and runs with them; it's his moment to shine and he's not about to let it go to waste.

It is utterly frustrating to see how many people get lost in desperation and continue to listen to the enemy. It is a critical stage, during which we should obviously reach out towards our Savior, yet so few seem to. How much healthier and happier could we be if only we made the choice to bask in God's warmth and love rather than the devil's trickery and confections? No matter how desperate your situation may seem, it is never more than God can handle. Reach out to the Lord for help so you can avoid the next part of Satan's cycle.

Gluttony

You've been craving hot wings and French fries all week long. To reward yourself for not giving in right away, you make plans to go out with friends. At the restaurant, you order twice as much as you normally eat, inhale everything, and decide to order seconds. Once our mind has been under bombardment by constant obsession and extreme desperation it almost always inevitably leads to gluttony. We tried to resist temptation for so long that once we give in and start eating, we can't seem to stop ourselves. We end up gorging, often to the point of illness. Gluttony is not looked upon favorably in the bible; it is evidence that we give in to temptation and sin over and over again. When you're in the gluttonous stage, you must realize that the enemy is winning the battle. He has gotten you completely distracted with harmful food. God wants to help us, but we need to turn to Him rather than a pan full of brownies.

Sadly, gluttony seems to be lauded in modern times. Everything seems to revolve around bigger being better. Restaurants typically increase their portion sizes to attract more customers and soft drinks are sold in containers large enough for a small infant to swim in. The devil has led us to demand more for our dollar, but sadly it has been in quantity rather than quality. We need to reverse the trend of overindulgence. The bible states in Proverbs 23:1-3, *"When you sit down to eat with a ruler, consider carefully what is before you; and put a knife to your throat if you are a man given to appetite. Do not desire his delicacies for they are deceptive food."* A bit drastic, yes, but we do need to sit up and take notice. If you are prone to excessive eating, it is time to stop. Simply because an abundance of food is available does not mean we should consume it. A knife to your throat causes pain and death, surely the bible would not direct us to inflict such agony upon ourselves—and yet, do you not realize a spoonful of junk food does the same thing? With every forkful of garbage you repeatedly place into your mouth you are inflicting horrendous damage internally. Ask God's forgiveness for your gluttonous ways and pray for His assistance to help you stop. Rest assured He will provide relief, for Proverbs 2:10-12 tells us, *"When wisdom enters your heart, and knowledge is pleasant to your soul, discretion will preserve you; understanding will keep you, to deliver you from the way of evil."*

Guilt

Immediately following a binging session, we are hit with a wave of guilt or disgust. We feel bad about not being stronger, not resisting the urge, giving in once again, and eating too much junk. It is quite easy to mistakenly believe that guilt is God's way of punishing us, of letting us know that we made the wrong choice and we should have known better. It is critical to know that guilt does not come from God. God will help make us aware of what is right and wrong, but He will not make us feel bad enough to punish ourselves. Look to 2 Corinthians 7:10 for further explanation, *"For godly sorrow produces repentance leading to salvation, not to be regretted; but the sorrow of the world produces death."* Guilt, or worldly sorrow, is yet another ploy cleverly used by the enemy. It is meant to bring you down and keep you down. Worldly sorrow can also show up in the form of vanity, in which we feel bad or self-conscious about our physical appearance. Regardless of the type of worldly sorrow, it produces the same result, which is spiritual separation from the Father. Godly sorrow, on the other hand, is when we know we are in the wrong and need to apologize and fix the situation. It's a much more positive way to deal with a problem and allows you the opportunity to own it and rectify it, which actually brings you a sense of empowerment rather than helplessness. The devil, however, just wants you to feel bad.

When we feel guilty about overeating, we tend to beat ourselves up mentally. We can be self-deprecating, miserable, angry, and much too hard on ourselves; these unconstructive thoughts and feelings do nothing except keep us in a spiritually stagnant place. We cannot be dejected and joyous simultaneously. It is hypocritical to praise our Creator, yet loathe ourselves. When you criticize yourself, you are critiquing God's work. Instead of letting the enemy fill our minds with thoughts of inferiority and feelings of worthlessness, we need to accept the fact that we are not flawless but we can strive towards perfection. We must first accept our culinary indiscretions and quickly move on. 2 Corinthians 7:11 provides hope, *"For observe this very thing, that you sorrowed in a godly manner: What diligence it produced in you, what clearing of yourselves, what indignation, what fear, what vehement desire, what zeal, what vindication!"* Let go of the negative guilt and instead embrace godly sorrow, which will empower you with the strength and motivation to overcome.

Denial

Denial is a popular defense mechanism that seems to have been invented by the devil himself. When a problem becomes so out of control and so unbearable that we can no longer accept it as a reality, a very serious problem is present. After guilt has eaten us from the inside out, we subconsciously turn to denial as a means of mental survival. Denying that a problem exists helps to ease the tremendous amount of guilt we're feeling and sends us off to a delusional "happy place." We deceive ourselves about many different things, despite the fact that these inconsistencies will always find their way to the surface. Following are some common delusions:

<u>"I'm not that fat."</u>

Few people actually seem to have an accurate idea of what their body type really is; typically, people are on two opposite sides of the spectrum. There are those individuals who are frighteningly underweight or even at an ideal weight, yet they are somehow convinced they are overweight. There are others who are morbidly obese, yet they can look in the mirror and not see themselves as fat. It is frightening to realize that there are people who are homebound, forced to shop in specialty clothing sizes, winded after walking up a flight of stairs, and told to their faces by a medical professional that they need to lose weight or they will die, yet they fail to come to face the reality of how unhealthy they truly are. The devil has a death hold on these individuals and does his best to keep them shielded from the truth. It is critical to understand and acknowledge the problem in order to overcome it. If you know someone who is obese, tell them. If someone is telling you to lose weight, listen. Take heed to what we are told in Matthew 18:18-20, *"Assuredly, I say to you, whatever you bind on earth will be bound in heaven, and whatever you loose on earth will be loosed in heaven. Again I say to you that if two of you agree on earth concerning anything that they ask, it will be done for them by My Father in heaven. For where two or three are gathered together in My name, I am there in the midst of them."*

"It could be worse."

Are there worse things you could be eating? Of course. Are there people who eat more poorly than you? No doubt. Just because you're not being as bad as you can does not equate to you being good. The devil will trick us into believing that our actions are justified by the fact that there are always worse choices we could be making. Ordering the small onion rings with your thrice-dipped in gravy beef sandwich does not mean you made a wise and nutritious selection; don't be swindled into believing otherwise. The key is to focus on your own continual self-improvement; you should never settle for less than your best self. For the same reasons that it is no good to compare yourself to the vegan marathoner-yogi down the street, it is of no benefit to compare yourself with the beer guzzling, donut eating couch potato on the next block either. Concentrate on your own battle and ways to win your war.

<u>"I don't mind being big."</u>

It seems some people have simply accepted themselves as being large and have tried to embrace it. It may seem like this is a good thing for positive self-image and self-love, but in reality it's just another trick of the enemy's. Being duped into believing that you should settle for a quality of life below what you can and deserve to have will only come from the devil. Even if being big is who you are, it's not who you have to be; inside of you is a person who is able to run or walk and who can make it through the day without back and knee pain. It is possible for you to have the energy and stamina to enjoy activities or play with your kids. Don't resolve yourself to a lifetime of pastries because the devil is telling you that you are destined to be large.

<u>"I'll do better next week."</u>

A popular lie we tell ourselves over and over again is that we will take charge of our cravings and eat healthier—tomorrow. Most, if not all, of you have told yourself this fib and you are well aware of how seldom it becomes true. We pick a date in the near future—next week, next month, after the holidays are over—and we decide that will be the first day of our new and improved self. Without fail, this magical day comes and goes just as every other day, and the only difference is that we're actually a pound or so heavier than we used to be.

There is an extreme danger with this line of thinking that stems from the misconception that we are in control. The simple fact is that God is in control. The enemy will delude you into thinking that you have the power and can dictate the way things play out on your own. Believing that you can gain control by yourself is the biggest lie people fall for and ultimately, it is what prevents success. The truth is that God is in control and unless your temptations are given over to Him, next week will be no better than the previous weeks.

<u>"My doctor hasn't told me I'm unhealthy."</u>

With the ever increasing number of people who are overweight, it has become acceptable to be fat. We see so many large people we have become desensitized and tend to forget how unhealthy they actually are. Weight is a sensitive issue for many people and it isn't easy to discuss openly, for this reason a lot of individuals simply avoid it, including some health professionals. Don't wait and rely on someone to inform you that you're at an unhealthy weight. Bring the topic up if your doctor fails to and figure out together what is a healthy weight range for you. Utilizing bandages and medications to alleviate symptoms of weight related issues, rather than dealing with the true cause is nothing more than a huge disservice to you.

Physical Pain and Death

More and more people are enduring needless suffering. There are aches and pains we feel on a regular basis that our bodies find a way to adapt to and there are issues going on below our skin's surface that we may not become aware of until it is too late. Thanks to modern medicine, many symptoms of obesity can be dealt with, giving us the illusion that the problem is gone. If you develop knee pain because your joints are unable to bear the burden of your weight, you can opt for surgery to repair it. If you become diabetic you can rely on insulin shots or pills. Drugs will also help lower blood pressure and cholesterol, and there are various medications to help ease difficulties with breathing. There is no medical cure for obesity and its side effects, there are simply means to make them more tolerable. Unfortunately, when the aches and pains are dulled it becomes easy to ignore the fact that there is still a large problem at hand. If you become stuck in this ocean of denial, your body simply deteriorates at a rapid pace until there is no turning back. As diseases get the best of your body, medications no longer work and doctors run out of procedures to perform. Symptoms pile on top of each other as your body shuts down. Loved ones are rendered helpless and must bear witness as you painstakingly approach your inevitable death.

Much of the needless suffering can be avoided. True, we will all die one day, but we do not have to sit idly by, pumping our bodies full of new chemicals to counter balance the years' worth of old chemicals we chewed up and swallowed time and again. Take this day to realize who it is you are at war with and prepare to arm yourself and fight, rather than succumb to a lifestyle riddled with pain and suffering.

"Finally, my brethren, be strong in the Lord and in the power of His might. Put on the whole armor of God, that you may be able to stand against the wiles of the devil. For we do not wrestle against flesh and blood, but against principalities, against powers, against the rulers of the

darkness of this age, against spiritual hosts of wickedness in the heavenly places. Therefore take up the whole armor of God, that you may be able to withstand in the evil day, and having done all, to stand.

Stand, therefore, having girded your waist with truth, having put on the breastplate of righteousness, and having shod your feet with the preparation of the gospel of peace; above all, taking the shield of faith with which you will be able to quench all the fiery darts of the wicked one. And take the helmet of salvation, and the sword of the Spirit, which is the word of God; praying always with all prayer and supplication in the Spirit, being watchful to this end with all perseverance and supplication for all the saints," Ephesians 6:10-18.

CHAPTER 4

BANISHING THE ENEMY FROM YOUR TEMPLE

"Do not destroy with your food the one for whom Christ died," Romans 14:15.

When you look in the mirror, what do you see? Do you focus on the cellulite accumulating around your thighs? Frightened by the bags under your eyes? Do you cringe at the flab on your upper arms? Disappointed by your soft, saggy middle? Too often our imperfections jump out at us. What about the fact that your legs make it possible for you to walk around? Aren't you amazed at the intricacies of your irises and all the beautiful things your eyes allow you to see? Don't forget those arms make it possible for you to squeeze your loved ones and that your core encases all of your vital organs that keep you living and breathing on this earth.

You need to start seeing your body for the temple that it is, no matter what shape you're in today. God created you; you are a work of God, His design, His sculpture, a piece of His art. How do you treat your temple, God's masterpiece? Are you defacing it by allowing extra pounds to accumulate? Do you dirty it up by letting junk flow through your arteries? Is the enemy helping you to graffiti your temple and turn it into a run-down mess?

If you think of your physical body not as your own, but rather as God's intricate design, wouldn't you treat it a bit differently? Perhaps you would think twice about imbibing high fructose corn syrup into your temple; maybe you would hold off on stuffing down unnecessary calories. The bible makes it clear in 2 Corinthians 6:16, *"For you are the temple of the living God."* There is no room for error or doubt in that statement, your body is most certainly a temple. Can it be made any more evident that your body is a shrine, worthy of being treated as such? In case simply knowing your body is a temple isn't enough to make you appreciate its sacredness, let's take it one step further. The bible states in 1 Corinthians 6:19-20, *"Do you not know that your body is the temple of the Holy Spirit who is in you, whom you have from God and you are not your own? For you were bought at a price; therefore, glorify God in your body and in your spirit, which are God's.*" Christ died a vicious death on the cross after enduring inhumane torture. As horrendous and humiliating as the death of Jesus Christ was, it served a greater purpose; He was sacrificed for you and me. He died a painful death to allow us opportunities and forgiveness. If you would pause to reflect on the gravity of His death on the cross for you, perhaps that might make you think twice about how you are treating His temple.

In Romans 14:15 we are given a direct order, "*Do not destroy with your food the one for whom Christ died.*" Rather than consuming unhealthy foods that bring us further from experiencing true joy and vitality, we should be eating in a way that uplifts and edifies. "*Therefore, whether you eat or drink, or whatever you do, do all to the glory of God,*" 1 Corinthians 10:31. Choose foods that would serve to glorify God. Eat in moderation to enjoy culinary creations, do not simply wallow in gluttony because an overabundance of food is readily available. You must realize the blessedness of your body, God's temple, and prepare yourself to eat and drink in a way that exalts our heavenly Father. Make it a focal point, not only as you continue reading, but in your everyday life. To truly defeat Satan, it will take a change in your thought patterns. You must view your body for what it actually is—a physical representation of God's temple. It is imperative that you begin to care for your body in the way God has entrusted you to do. Don't waste another negative moment hating your body, resenting parts or criticizing it. Your body, no matter the size or shape it is in today, is an astonishing machine built in such intricate detail that even the most intelligent scientists and medical professionals cannot fully comprehend all of its inner workings. You need to strive to make any and all improvements you can. Get your holy place as clean and polished as possible.

You should want it to sparkle and shine and be in top-notch form because you do have an appointment to one day meet your Maker.

Now that you realize how important your body is, how do you go about incorporating food into your spiritual life? The concept of eating and drinking in a positive, joyful, and reverent manner pertains heavily to when we are gathered with friends and family. Feasting with others should be a time of fellowship and it is even an opportunity to worship. "*So continuing daily with one accord in the temple, and breaking bread from house to house, they ate their food with gladness and simplicity of the heart, praising God and having favor with all the people. And the Lord added to the church daily those who were being saved,*" Acts 2:46-47. Jesus certainly knew how to throw a party, He made sure food was readily available and was even known to turn water into wine. It wasn't the food and drink that made the celebration, however, it was the company. Their focus was on the companionship, camaraderie, and teachings with the bread and wine thrown in as an added bonus. We need to revert back to simpler times when the importance was less on the dishes being served and more on the conversations being initiated. Sharing a meal with someone is a time to commune and the focus should be on togetherness. Sadly, many electronics such as television, smartphones, and tablets have become regular guests during mealtimes and they are nothing more than major distractions. These devices can take away your concentration from those you are supposed to be enjoying your feast with and they can also divert you into mindless eating. Remove technology from the table and direct your efforts into establishing a mindful and spiritual presence instead.

The significance of breaking bread was established with the Lord's Supper, as written in Matthew 26:26, *"And as they were eating, Jesus took bread, blessed and broke it, and gave it to the disciples and said, 'Take, eat; this is My body.'"* Anyone who takes communion is familiar with the scenario of eating in remembrance of Jesus' sacrifice, but the breaking of bread is not something that should be confined to Sunday mornings in church. Have you ever literally broken bread with someone? If not, I suggest it. Put away your germaphobe tendencies, grab a hunk of bread with a loved one, and pull. Not only is it fun and playful, it immediately establishes a bond. It is hands-on sharing at a primal level that conveys love, acceptance, and comfort; and if that isn't God's plan for us as humans, I don't know what is.

How many of you, when sitting down to eat dinner, will recite a prayer and ask Him to bless to your body the food you are about to eat? What if you're about to consume a large stuffed pizza topped with pepperoni, sausage, and three types of cheese? Would that type of meal hold the same nutritional blessing as a colorful salad heaping with nuts, seeds, and veggies? Not likely, and it's insulting to God's intelligent design of things to think that they would even come close. God has granted us with free will and that includes the option to have the greasy, fattening meals once in a while. Perhaps we should do a better job of acknowledging this, though. To be honest, nearly anytime I sit down for a less than healthy meal and we ask for a blessing, I'll typically add on a mental, "Please do with this what you can, Lord." My added prayer is that He will allow my body to utilize whatever nutrients are in the meal and that the garbage will be efficiently filtered out. Also, if I notice that recent meals have been lacking in the beneficial department I'll ask for some divine help to correct that, ASAP. I encourage you to try those little tips and also to see if you can feel the difference in the blessing of a healthy meal versus an unhealthy one.

Start enjoying nutritious food for the pure, unadulterated nourishment that it is. Rejoice at mealtimes and delight in any company you may be blessed to eat with, rather than stressing over minute details. *"Better is a dinner of herbs where love is, than a fatted calf with hatred,"* Proverbs 15:17. Lastly, stop taking your body—your temple—for granted as you only get one.

CHAPTER 5
IN DEFENSE OF
CHOCOLATE

"But food does not commend us to God; for neither if we eat are we the better, nor if we do not eat are we the worse," 1 Corinthians 8:8.

Sugars and fats are inanimate objects, completely unable to defend themselves. As an avid lover of all things chocolate, I do feel the need to speak in defense of food everywhere, rather than suffer a lifelong feeling of disloyalty and dishonor every time I unwrap a cocoa confectionary. I am focusing on chocolate because it is something that I enjoy, but the truth is that whatever food it is that you personally savor will still pertain to the same idea. You can find nutrition in nearly any food when it's consumed in moderation. The opposite also holds true, however, in that you can find detrimental health effects in nearly every food when consumed in excess. Whatever food it is that makes your taste buds do a happy dance, simply find the right balance. Truthfully, it's not as hard as you think. When you finish eating your treat and you feel satisfied, happy, and good about it, you've consumed a decent amount. When you are left feeling guilty, bloated, stuffed, and ill or unsatisfied, you went overboard. Focus on relishing the food itself, not simply the amount. With a little prayer and self-control you can actually gain more satisfaction from eating less of your favorite treat.

To go one step further, try to find the most nutritional form of your chosen delicacy. My glorious day came when I unearthed the wonders of cacao powder, chocolate in its simplest and most pure form. Not only is it extremely versatile, it's full of antioxidants, polyphenols, fiber, magnesium, and other nutrients that are good for you, while, believe it or not, it contains none of the bad stuff. If cacao is actually healthy, how did we end up with so many candy bars full of fats and sugars containing little actual cacao? Do I think the candy man was in cahoots with the devil? No, probably not. Satan has a way of taking almost anything we like and exploiting it to exorbitant heights, turning something that was once merely enjoyable into an all-encompassing addiction. It's also a prime example of how the enemy manages to turn something that offers healthful benefits into an artery clogging grenade. The enemy uses his influence to inflict harm upon us in any way possible, all the more reason for you to be more vigilant and aware of what you are choosing to consume.

So how can you make your favorite food more nutritionally satisfying? First, don't be afraid to splurge in the appropriate way. My penchant for chocolate has evolved from that of a gluttonous child, eager to get her grubby hands on every available morsel of chocolate within sniffing distance, into a passionate cocoa connoisseur. I would rather indulge in an exotic, creamy, bold *piece* of chocolate than an entire bar comprised of inferior components. Yes, I am that person who would forgo a jumbo sized bag of inexpensive chocolate to pay the same price for a small bar made with high quality ingredients. I don't even balk at the price difference anymore because ounce for ounce, it's worth it. Spend the extra money because it will force you to slow down and savor the treat more. When we acquire things cheaply, they lose their value to us and that should not be the case when we are indulging ourselves. Not only does splurging slow you down and decrease the amount you consume, it typically guarantees you're putting higher quality ingredients into your body, thereby giving it greater nutritional value. A generic chocolate bar will typically contain sugar or corn syrups, milk fats, emulsifiers, and artificial flavors to name a few, and these don't offer much in terms of health. Take a look at what comprises a specialty chocolate bar, however, and suddenly you're looking at actual cocoa and all of its nutritional benefits. By modifying my choices, my favorite treat went from illness causing to illness preventing. Do a little research into your preferred food and find ways to enjoy it while benefiting your health. Anything that you can make from scratch yourself is sure to be better for you right off the bat. You know what ingredients are in it and it should not contain any chemical preservatives. There are less detrimental packaged food options as well, if that is the road you must take; spend a little time comparing ingredients or peruse the internet to find healthier substitutes because it is very much worth your while. It may cost a little more money than you're used to spending, but remember that you are worth it and so is the experience of enjoying your favorite delicacy, guilt and detriment free. Spending a little more time and money up front can also have huge savings in the long run in terms of health care for you, your family, and even society as a whole.

I want to share a personal story that I think exemplifies the art of savoring and moderation. I once went on a guided walking chocolate tour, and we were led to various chocolatiers throughout the city to sample some of their finest creations. As you can well imagine the samples were not large quantities, but the tour wasn't about gorging ourselves on as much chocolate as we could possibly stuff into our bellies. No, it was the experience of finding new chocolate boutiques we never knew existed and the adventure of trying cocoa paired with crazy ingredients you would never imagine marrying together. Given my predilection for savoring, I easily managed to turn a small truffle into four or five bites and thoroughly enjoyed each morsel. In comparison, at one point I watched a woman pop an entire truffle into her mouth in one shot. I would venture to say I gleaned way more satisfaction from nibbling mine. How can I be so certain? Simple math for starters; my three extra bites allowed me the opportunity to extend the flavor, relish it, and experience the varying tastes that exploded in my mouth at different points in time. Want further proof? She needed to purchase a whole box to take home to extend her pleasure. As for myself, I obtained enough satisfaction from one truffle that I didn't feel compelled to buy more, a bonus for my waist and wallet.

The bottom line is that foods themselves cannot be blamed for making you unhealthy. Sugar, fat, salt—or whatever your poison of choice—is not going to damage you. *Over-consumption* of any of these things will. It is perfectly fine to partake of your favorite delicacy on occasion and in reasonable amounts. The secret is to know who is in control and realize that God has provided the opportunity for you to enjoy this treat, so honor Him by taking time to truly relish the dish.

CHAPTER 6
GOING TO BATTLE

"Behold, I give you the authority to trample on serpents and scorpions, and over all the power of the enemy, and nothing shall by any means hurt you," Luke 10:19.

Satan is a formidable enemy; his evil knows no bounds and that is a frightening thought. Fortunately, he can be defeated. There is no question, the devil does not hold absolute power. The devil's plans can be thwarted, both on small and grand scale schemes; we are guaranteed that in the end, he will lose. Is it scary to think that the devil and his demons are attacking us on a daily basis, in our own familiar territory? Yes. Is it depressing to think that our health is suffering because we have allowed ourselves to be bested by Satan? Certainly. Does it seem an unnervingly daunting task to declare war against evil incarnate, the father of sin, and the one who instigated the fall of humanity? Without a doubt. So why on earth should you be expected to take on the army of darkness? Because—and this is important—if you choose to fight, you can be absolutely certain you will be triumphant. You are guaranteed victory, you cannot lose. You will succeed and defeat evil; the outcome has been decided. There is a winning team and a losing one, all you have to do is choose who you want to align yourself with. It really is that simple. You know who your real enemy is, now make the choice to stand against him and you will win. I don't want to sugar coat things too much; you will face difficulties, experience setbacks, and lose some battles. Just because you are certain to win the war doesn't mean everything will be handed to you, easy as pie. Knowing who holds the power should make every encounter a little easier for you to handle, though. Let's look at some ways to help you face down each struggle. First, I must warn you, if you're looking for a complex scheme with loads of intricate details, look elsewhere; if you want a diet plan, complete with weighing your food to properly measure your calories, it won't be found here. The way to defeat Satan is basic, simple, and dates back to the beginning of time. Will you experience challenges? Yes, but there is no such thing as an easy war.

Awareness

It might not seem like the most aggressive war tactic, but it is one of the most important. The point of this book is to make you conscious of your true enemy and the fact that he's been using something as familiar as food to sabotage you. As the saying goes, knowledge is power. You no longer have to waste time, energy, and emotions on aimlessly trying to beat the battle of the bulge by throwing efforts in all directions, hoping blindly that something will finally pay off and work. Declare war on the true enemy and let that be your focus.

Start by increasing your awareness whenever food is involved. Ask God to remove the scales from your eyes and allow you to see what is going on. Pay attention before, during, and after a meal. Notice when a craving strikes you—what it is, where you are, what's going on in your mind and around you. Watch what you choose to eat and how much you eat. Critique advertisements for food and drink, even make mental note when people offer you food. Before you take a bite, take a moment to pause and reflect on what you're about to put in your mouth. You can keep notes or a journal, if that helps you and there are countless apps to help you monitor your consumption. Your goal is to tune into the ways Satan and his minions are tempting you, teasing you, and attacking you. I am urging you to be aware. We have become so indifferent to unhealthy food bombardment around us, so used to seeing junk food every which way we turn, that it is now the norm and we have become utterly desensitized. Allow yourself no feelings of guilt and no passing judgment. Try to be an impartial observer and take an open and honest look at the food and beverage being presented or made available to you in your daily life.

Once you're aware of the devil's culinary attacks, you need to focus your attention on food itself. First of all, detach yourself from any emotions or thoughts pertaining to food, as it is inanimate. Food is simply something you put into your mouth that your body has to break down to utilize for nourishment or work to expel from your system. Food is not your friend, nor is it your foe. Remove the term "emotional eater" from your vocabulary, because food itself cannot bring you solace or comfort. Force yourself to be aware of food for exactly what it is. Stop letting Satan trick you into using your feelings as an excuse to eat more; don't listen to him when he tries to convince you that junk food is your crutch or that it will bring you unrelenting joy. Examine food for what it really is—sustenance, pure and simple. Fruits, veggies, healthy proteins, and grains will nourish your body so it can run properly, while junk food will clog things up and tax your system.

Once you can start to remove emotional value from food you can see Satan's attacks much more clearly. Just a warning—this part may sting a little. You've been enjoying food for years, it has been a constant companion and now you're faced with the black and white truth that you've been completely duped. As we all know, sometimes the truth hurts, even when it is for our own betterment. It's like finding out one day that your best friend has been secretly cavorting with your arch nemesis and they've been playing tricks on you for years behind your back. It's okay to hurt and be more than a little upset. Channel your anger because it is this fury that you should use to battle the enemy, but be sure to save it for the appropriate times, when you're ready for war. Right now you need to keep focus on your awareness and observations; you're on your reconnaissance mission, gathering information that is absolutely critical to your crusade. Figure out what he is tempting you with. How? Where does he strike? When does he strike? What people in your life is he using in order to get to you? Pay close attention and be extremely suspicious because there is no stooping too low for the devil, yet there is no scheme too grandiose for him either. He will not hesitate to work through your sweet old Grandma Betsy and he can all too easily pull off finagling his motives through even the largest fast food chain.

Prayer

Of all the things you can do in your quest to defeat evil, prayer is the single most powerful. I mentioned you can beat Satan, but I didn't say you could do it without help. Depending upon where you are at in your battle with weight, you will have a long, difficult journey ahead of you. Let's face it, this isn't just your run-of-the-mill bad guy. You are battling Satan, who is ultimately waging war for your soul. You're going to need all the help you can get.

Sadly it seems to be human nature for people to fall to their knees in helpless prayer when they are at the very end of their rope, when they have nowhere left to turn and they've run out of options. Why wait? So many people will turn to pills, diet fads, personal trainers, and doctors first. It's not until all of these professionals tell us there is nothing more they can do, until we are diagnosed with a life-threatening disease, until we realize that we are about to expire, that we finally turn to God for help. Kind of late in the game isn't it? The truth is, there is no need to wait to ask for help. Whether you're ten pounds over-weight or two hundred, if you are facing a struggle, you need to seek help and start praying immediately.

What if you're not quite sure how to pray? Pray about whatever is on your heart and mind. Start a conversation with God—tell Him your worries, concerns, hopes, and struggles, and most importantly, ask for His help, His guidance, and His protection. I'm not going to give you a specific prayer to repeat that only has meaning for me. You need to establish a prayerful life on your own terms, something that works for you. God wants to hear from you in your own voice, in your own words. He needs to know what's bothering you, what's hurting you, what's holding you back and how He can help. Make sure that you also pray for God to reveal the enemy and how he is operating in your life. You need to know where the demons are hiding and how they are attacking you so you can prepare yourself to battle them. I know battling evil may seem daunting, even downright frightening, but you need to know so you can move forward. Remember that you are not alone and victory is on your side.

When should you pray? Whenever you need to! Pray for knowledge before meals to make proper choices, pray for strength during meals to know when to stop. Pray whenever you experience a craving, anytime food pops into your mind you can ask God to remove the temptation. Pray before you go into a grocery store, a restaurant, or any type of social event where food is featured. Pray when you're planning a meal, if you're not sure what to eat, and pray when you want to eat something you know you shouldn't. Prayer is your single most powerful weapon, use it as much as you possibly can. *"Ask, and it will be given to you; seek, and you will find; knock, and it will be opened to you. For everyone who asks receives, and he who seeks finds, and to him who knocks it will be opened,"* Matthew 7:7-8.

Control

For a long time, Satan has been wielding control of your fork. He's been guiding you to shovel unhealthy garbage down your gullet for years. He's seen you through every over-indulgence, every late night craving, and every sugar coma you've partaken in. You have let him influence you for far too long and must now face the consequences. Some might believe this to be impossible, they think the devil has no sway over what we do. Then why is it that we can't seem to put our fork down although we know we've eaten enough? Why do we eat three-quarters of a bag of potato chips before we even think about slowing down? Why is it so imperative to finish all the food on our behemoth-sized plate? Why do we stock cupboards with food that is doing more harm than good? Why do we repeatedly eat convenient foods in lieu of nutritious, yet satisfying foods? Why do we accept seconds or refills even though we've supposedly committed to a diet? Who in their right mind would choose a life of pain and suffering, wrought with never ending struggles? No one would consciously opt for this type of lifestyle, yet millions of us are living it, every day because we've elected to follow Satan's food deceptions. Have no doubt, Satan's MO is to tempt us with instant pleasure and gratification, but it is always accompanied by deferred pain.

Immediately, you must regain control from Satan and his demons. Take back your power of eating—stop believing his lies and deceit. Once you've reclaimed control of your diet from the devil, relinquish it to God. Give it up completely, right away. Ask God for His help in determining what you should eat, as well as the quantity. Ask God to fill your plate, to write your grocery list, to lead you to healthy and tasty new recipes. Put the reins where they belong for your own preservation. Have no doubt in your mind that God will gladly provide you with the appropriate amount you need. We can look to Exodus 16 for an enlightening example. *"And Moses said to them, 'This is the bread which the Lord had given you to eat. This is the thing which the Lord has commanded: "Let every man gather it according to each one's need, one omer for each person, according to the number of persons; let every man take for those who are in his tent."'*

Then the children of Israel did so and gathered, some more, some less. So when they measured it by omers, he who gathered much had nothing left over, and he who gathered little had no lack. Every man had gathered according to each one's need. And Moses said, 'Let no one leave any of it till morning.' Notwithstanding they did not heed Moses. But some of them left part of it until morning, and it bred worms and stank,"* Exodus 16:15-20. If you read the entire chapter you will learn that God was testing the people's faith in His provisions as well as their own ability to follow His instructions. Learn from their mistake, as well as your own and start relying on God's perfect provision for your needs.

Ditch the Diet Plans

No-carb, low-carb, fat free, sugar free, fruit diets, detox diets, location based diets—there have been so many diet plans pimped out in the last few decades it's enough to make your head spin. Combine all these fad diets with trying to decipher nutrition labels and listen to various experts telling you what to look for, what to avoid, how much to include, how much to exclude and it's no wonder people give up and do their grocery shopping based on pretty pictures.

The vast majority of all diet plans and nutrition fads are nothing more than a Trojan horse. It's simply the devil presenting you with a package, a plan, or a means to success that once you accept does nothing more than ultimately lead to further destruction. Most of the diet industry is based on a mirage, an illusion, a fallacy. It's a way of preying on the desperate to make money selling false hopes and dreams. True, there are some success stories for every diet-related pitch available, but the recognition should go to the individuals who were able to lose the weight rather than the method itself. I think it has much more to do with their own personal faith, commitment, and perseverance than anything else. You must be aware of these Trojan horse diet fads. When you learn about a new diet craze, be skeptical, be hesitant, and don't jump into it with both eyes closed. You should do research and pray about it before starting any new diet plan. Find out if it is something God would have you follow. If not, look elsewhere.

Extreme diets can cause damage to your body on a physiological level. Starving yourself on a meager calorie diet may help you shed a few pounds relatively quickly, but at a cost. Denying your body sustenance will create an imbalance and it will naturally go into survival mode to compensate. Almost anyone who has attempted any form of starvation can undoubtedly attest to the fact that you end up gaining more weight back than the few pounds initially lost. Do you need to cut calories? Almost certainly, yes, but you should not restrict your caloric intake to the point that it taxes your body simply to function at a basic level.

Don't forget to take into account the psychological harm that fad diets can have on a person either. How many times have you excitedly started a new diet plan convinced that you were turning over a new leaf, ready to become a whole new healthier you, certain of success this time, only to find yourself floundering and reverting back to old habits? How many times have you stuck to a weight-loss plan for days, weeks, maybe even months before you gave up because you weren't obtaining the promised results? When you attempt to follow a fad diet, you're setting yourself up for failure. Trendy diets don't work, and that is why they are popular for only a limited amount of time. Think of the damage done to your morale when you fail at yet another diet attempt. How guilty do you feel? How much self-punishment do you inflict, even at a sub-conscious level? How long does it take you to get back on the horse and restart your quest for health? These are all factors that harm your psyche, your body, and your spirit.

Rather than latch on to a trendy diet, you would be much better off to learn how to eat what your body needs. Learn a little about nutrition, spend some time finding out just how those fruits, veggies, proteins, and good fats can fuel your body, helping you to function at a more optimal level. You don't need to pursue a degree in nutrition, but a little bit of knowledge will go a long way in helping you make better food choices. When you learn of all the vitamins, minerals, antioxidants, and fiber packed into one apple it just might take your respect for the mundane fruit to a whole new level. On the flip side, when you learn of all the cancer and disease causing ingredients in processed foods it will hopefully make you rethink a candy bar for a snack. Don't just blindly follow another diet plan in hopes that it will work, empower yourself. Having the knowledge will give you confidence to make wise food choices, and I'm sure you'll quickly realize that you already know how to eat healthy, or at least have some idea. It comes down to you forcibly removing the blinders that Satan has put on you and no longer following his duplicity.

I know some of you may need to follow a diet plan, especially in the beginning and that's perfectly okay. Just make sure that you pick a plan that makes sense and doesn't leave you starving. Your diet should include vegetables, fruits, proteins, healthy fats, and plenty of water. Don't follow anything that sounds to gimmicky or too good to be true, because most likely it is. There are plenty of options available that will allow you to eat healthy and be satisfied. Be sure to pray for God's wisdom and guidance when choosing your nutritional foundation and don't be afraid to seek assistance, spiritual or professional, when you need it.

Learn to Recognize Help

God will send help your way and it's important that you are ready to acknowledge it, as it will bolster your spirit to continue fighting. It's critical that you keep your eyes and heart open to God's form of help. Rarely does He work in over-the-top dramatic miracles. You will most likely not suddenly find sugary sweets distasteful, pounds will not magically shed off you overnight, and you won't start craving salads before bedtime, but that does not mean He is ignoring your pleas for help. How God will assist you personally I cannot say, but I can list some possibilities.

God often sends help in human form. People you may already know, or new people you encounter may be working on the Lord's behalf. Maybe it's a physician, who has mentioned you can relieve some of your symptoms if you lose weight. Perhaps God is sending you assistance through friends and family members who offer encouragement. Support groups, dietitians, pastors, teachers, even children can be vessels of God, delivering you strength, support, knowledge or anything you might need. Don't discount anyone who takes an interest in your health and diet, as Hebrews 13:2 tells us, *"Do not forget to entertain strangers, for by so doing some have unwittingly entertained angels."*

Although the media is constantly bombarding us with negativity, it is safe to assume that God uses this channel for His own purposes as well. It can be very difficult, however, to decipher His message from that of the enemy and so we must be extremely wary of what we see and hear in mainstream media. Various television shows, from the news to documentaries or talk shows, will offer health and wellness tips. There are magazines dedicated solely to improved health, and most other magazines will, at the very least, include articles on the subject. There is a plethora of books that have been written about nutrition and well-being. The task we face is to determine what information is Godly and what is polished up garbage from Satan. You should rely on prayer for this undertaking and rely upon the Lord to guide you. Eventually you'll start to see proper nutrition is mostly common sense. God has provided us with nourishment and the more you consume natural foods, the better. As Psalm 104:14-15 states, *"He causes the grass to grow for the cattle, and vegetation for the service of man, that he may bring forth food from the earth, and wine that makes glad the heart of man, oil to make his face shine, and bread which strengthens man's heart."* The quickest, easiest way to determine bogus information from beneficial is to hold strong and fast to the belief that if it *comes from* a plant *of* the Earth, it's more than likely good for you, but if it was *created in* a plant, it's more than likely not.

Lastly, to grasp the full concept of this book, we must believe that spiritual warfare is real and is going on around us. If the devil and his demons are against us, it would stand to reason that we have an army of angels as our allies, and we are promised as much in the bible. *"For He shall give His angels charge over you, to keep you in all your ways,"* Psalm 91:11. I cannot go into detail in regards to angels because I simply do not know. I do believe the spiritual realm exists around us, but it remains a mystery to me and is way beyond the scope of this book. At this point, I hope it is enough comfort for you to know that God's angels are fighting for you and will help you in your battles. Find comfort in Psalm 103:20, *"Bless the Lord, you His angels, who excel in strength, who do His word, heeding the voice of His word."* I urge you to look for the handiwork of angels and maintain faith in their good works during your struggles. If angels presented themselves to assist Jesus, as seen in Matthew 4:11, *"Then the devil left Him, and behold, angels came and ministered to Him,"* certainly we can count on them to come to our aid as well.

Relish the Small Victories

Realize that you are fully engaged in warfare. Depending on the strength of Satan's grasp over your nutrition, it will be a series of difficult battles. Obviously you're familiar with the struggle by now, as you've been dealing with it for years. However, the tide has turned—you will now be going to battle fully aware of what is happening and conscious of the fact that Satan and his demons are simply trying to engorge you into misery. Celebrating your victories over Satan and his demons will help empower you to continue. Every time you refuse junk food, each time you say no to un-healthy fodder you must realize your victory and stand a little taller. For every single pound you lose and every soda you pass on, acknowledge your own strength and determi-nation. You will face multiple temptations on a daily basis, especially in the beginning of your journey because the enemy does not want to see you gain positive momentum. It will be a constant uphill battle against any and all culinary temptations. The good news is that the mountain isn't nearly as tall as it seems. You fight, you claw, you scramble your way through those battles, dodging and deflect-ing with everything you've got and rely on the

Lord to take over when you can't. It will be dirty, dark, and ugly. There will be setbacks and new challenges you never would have expected, problems that seem insurmountable at times, but you *can* do it. Satan fights dirty and unfair, but ultimately, God prevails.

It is difficult, on a day to day basis to keep your eyes on the bigger picture and that is why it is so crucial to bask in the glow of even the smallest of accomplishments. It does you no good to feel bad or focus on failures, which is merely smack talk from the enemy camp. So if you had one cookie instead of three, if you chose a healthy breakfast over sugary cereal, or if you skipped the side of fries, rejoice. Let each and every one of your triumphs, no matter how small they may seem, bolster your confidence and propel you to continue making wise decisions and ignoring the demons. Satan will hate you for it. In all of your euphoria and celebrating, make sure you don't forget praise; praise and glory go to God, for He is making all things possible. Give yourself a small pat on the back, but be sure to bow your head and give thanks and credit where it is due.

CHAPTER 7

FIGHTING FOR OTHERS

"Therefore, if food makes my brother stumble, I will never again eat meat, lest I make my brother stumble," 1 Corinthians 8:13.

There is an important issue that needs to be addressed. It is a sensitive topic and could easily offend. If you are an overweight or obese parent, it is very likely that your children are, or soon will be suffering from a weight issue as well. I feel the need to speak the truth. My intent is not to harm, belittle, ridicule, or anything of the sort. My goal is the complete opposite, so if you are the parent of an overweight child, please put down your hackles. Please do not go into overprotective overdrive, please open your eyes, your ears, and your heart because your child's life depends on it. I would never attack the worth, the value, or the integrity of a child and I am not questioning your love or skills as a parent.

Childhood obesity is on the rise at an alarmingly high rate. Today's children run the risk of dying before their parents and I hate the thought of any parent having to bury their child, especially for something that is preventable. No mom wants to imagine endless trips to the doctors for her son and no dad can stand the thought of his daughter facing a lifetime dependency on drugs for a life-threatening medical condition. Some parents don't have a choice, but many of us do. Many children are unhealthy simply because of a poor diet and lack of exercise and we, as parents, need to change that. Why do so many loving parents allow their children to be unhealthy? It's so easy to see injuries in the form of cuts, bruises, and scrapes, but what about the physical harm being done to the obese child? We cannot see the organs struggling to function due to accumulated visceral fat, we can't see the thickened arteries, the heart struggling to pump, but that doesn't mean it's not happening.

I have seen overweight children being pulled around in wagons, pushed in strollers with their feet dragging on the ground, huffing while walking up stairs, and enticed to complete sports classes with promises of ice cream right after. How are we serving these children? We aren't. Parents, by not making healthy choices for your children, you are accelerating their physical and spiritual death while setting them up for a lifetime of medical problems. Friends, family, teachers, and coaches, by turning a blind eye you are allowing children to suffer needlessly. The fight for our children's health is a crucial one. It is one that will not go unrewarded, as Jesus promises us in Mark 9:37, *"Whoever receives one of these little children in My name receives Me; and whoever receives not Me, but Him who sent Me."*

Matthew 10:42 states, *"And whoever gives one of these little ones only a cup of cold water in the name of a disciple, assuredly, I say to you, he shall by no means lose his reward."* Upon first glance, giving a little one only a cup of cold water sounds so meager, almost cheap and stingy. In our society, given the ease at which we can access juice, soda, sports drinks, and vitamin waters for our kids, anyone who's merely providing some water is pretty tightfisted. Why not go above and beyond by serving them a more flavorful beverage? Give them the sugar they crave, give them what tastes good. That's probably your initial reaction to reading the above verse, right? What if you read it with a slightly different perspective?

Without water, we will die. Our bodies are made up primarily of water and bodily functions rely on it. We need water. Water is life. We do not need water mixed with sugars, food colorings, corn syrups, and natural flavorings. In fact, all of these extra ingredients only serve to clog up and slow down our body's ability to operate. When you give a child *only* a cup of water, you are giving them only what they need, only what their body craves. You are not bogging them down with artificial junk. You are improving their body, their health, their quality of life. Giving a child *only* a cup of water is far more loving and generous than giving a child any sort of sweetened chemical elixir.

Of course, this train of thought pertains to everything you provide a child to consume. Giving a child an actual orange is far more generous than allowing them to eat an orange flavored ice pop. We need to be careful to not fall into the devil's trap that we must buy children junk as treats. We should not be lured into imbibing our kids with sugars and chemicals because of colorful packaging or the cartoon characters telling us to do so. I know it can be highly tempting when their eyes light up and excited hops are punctuated by squeals of delight, but we must not forget it is our job to protect these precious little ones. We know their lives are sought after by the evil one and it is our responsibility to be aware of the enemy's attacks on our children. Obviously this will require a massive shift in your thought process, as we have been convinced for years that indulging a child shows love. You are correct in predicting that changing their food options will come with a lot of complaint and defiance, but parents and caregivers, I urge you to stand your ground for the sake of the child. Don't underestimate our kids, they inherently want to do what is right and if you teach them about eating for their body's benefit they will want to do it. *"Behold, children are a heritage from the Lord, the fruit of the womb is a reward,"* Psalm 127:3. Whatever the short term ramifications, it is vital that we get our children on a healthy path.

The war on obesity is obviously not limited to children and our attempts to help should not be restricted to kids. Granted, it is much harder to tell a grown up what to eat, but there are things we can do to help our brothers and sisters. The first, and probably most obvious form of assistance would be to pray for them. Once again, prayer is intimate and personal and I am not a fan of pre-worded prayers so I will not use these pages to create a generic prayer for you to recite. Instead, I encourage you to speak what's on your heart and begin your own dialogue with God. Raise your concerns and ask Him how you can assist others.

In addition to prayer, we are called to be more proactive and take action to aid others. One practical thing we can do is to modify our behavior around others. 1 Corinthians chapter 8 gives an explanation that Christians can eat foods that were offered to idols because we know that idols mean nothing. If your friend shares with you a pot roast she originally offered up to her golden calf you are still free to partake because you know her statue is nothing more than a hunk of metal. The problem, however, is the example you're setting for others who aren't aware. Maybe your friend invited her sister to dinner as well and now she thinks that her calf-worshipping sister has converted the Christian, or, at the very least, found a weakness in the lining of the believer's stomach. We must be mindful of our behavior, for even if we know the true meaning and motive, others may not. Thankfully, dedicating meals to idols isn't as common place anymore, but do not let your guard down for even a moment. If the devil and his demons have been lurking in your kitchen, they most certainly will be hanging out in those of your friends and family. Even if you've banished the devil from your pantry, others more than likely aren't privy to his presence. When they witness what could be labeled "bad" behavior or poor eating habits without knowing the underlying motive, they become even more susceptible to the lies.

The bible tells us in 1 Corinthians 8:12-13, *"When you sin against the brethren and wound their weak conscience, you sin against Christ. Therefore, if food makes my brother stumble, I will never again eat meat, lest I make my brother stumble,"* and in Romans

15:1-2, *"We then who are strong ought to bear with the scruples of the weak, and not to please ourselves. Let each of us please his neighbor for his good, leading to edification."* These verses of scripture make it pretty clear that we are given a huge amount of responsibility. When you enjoy unhealthy treats, even if you're doing it free from sin, free from Satan's influence, you still have an obligation to avoid those foods for your brother's sake. You must set an example, otherwise you're helping the enemy. If you don't abstain from treats when others are around you who are deeply entwined in Satan's grasp, you are only furthering his evil cause. It's not always easy to pass by the dessert table simply for the benefit of others, but it is something we are called to do. The bible further reiterates this point in Romans 14:20-22, *"Do not destroy the work of God for the sake of food. All things indeed are pure, but it is evil for the man who eats with offense. It is good neither to eat meat nor drink wine nor do anything by which your brother stumbles or is offended or is made weak. Do you have faith? Have it to yourself before God."* As the verse—and common sense—tells us that it's not a good idea to toss back a few cold ones with an alcoholic, why do we think it's okay to share a pie with someone who is obese? How can we expect them to curb their appetite if we can't exemplify discipline ourselves? When you know someone is being beaten down by the enemy, it seems very cruel to offer goodies and treats that aren't healthy. If you have given control of your food consumption over to God, look at Romans 14:22 as a reminder to partake in the less healthy fare while you are not in the presence of an individual who is struggling. When you are free from Satan's culinary control over you, there is still more work to be done. You must be strong for your neighbors, don't drag them into temptation. Don't let them think for a moment that Satan gets the best of you through junk food. There should be no brownie gooey enough to entice you to play a part in the destruction of one of God's creations. Eat healthy in an edifying way in their company and know that there is a time and place for you to enjoy food purely for the pleasure. That time should include reverence and praise, not coercion and guilt. *"Brethren, if a man is overtaken in any trespass, you who are spiritual restore such a one in a spirit of gentleness, considering yourself lest you also be tempted. Bear one another's burdens, and so fulfill the law of Christ,"* Galatians 6:1-2.

You already know how much Satan enjoys a good party. When you are hosting an event, do your best to make it a healthy one. Forgo the burgers and dogs and offer a healthy variety instead. If you're not the host, be sure to bring a nutritious side dish. In no time at all, it will become a standing tradition that you can be counted on to bring a fruit or veggie entrée. Will comments be made? Yes, definitely. People will grumble, but take peace in the knowledge that you are fighting on their behalf in a war they may not even be aware of. In addition, a lot of people actually love trying a new dish, especially if it's good for them. Make sure it's something yummy and be prepared to share your recipe, because nearly everyone loves to add a healthy new dish to their repertoire. I hope you realize what a chain reaction you have the potential to enact. Simply abandoning the comfort and convenience of unhealthy traditions can have an incalculable impact on your loved ones and their loved ones.

Lastly, when you fight, do so with the strength of compassion, acceptance, and love. Love is truly your strongest artillery when battling for someone else. No one responds well to harsh judging, criticizing, insulting, or belittling. You must have empathy and understanding. You must not forget that your unhealthy loved one is a prisoner of war. *"Let brotherly love continue. . . . Remember the prisoners as if chained with them—those who are mistreated since you yourselves are in the body also,"* Hebrews 13:1-3. We should treat the afflicted with love. Don't parade your skinny new self around, insist that your way is the only way, and never even think about casting them off. Rather, we should tell them the truth. Let them know they are in a battle with the devil, that he wants them overweight and miserable. Then pray for them, pray with them, whatever they need. You simply, purely, and truly love them.

Because the word of God is more powerful than anything I could ever print, I want to leave you with scripture. The following verses are your playbook in fighting Satan's food war for the sake of others:

"If your brother is grieved because of your food, you are no longer walking in love," Romans 14:15.

"Owe no one anything except to love one another, for he who loves another has fulfilled the

law," Romans 13:8.

"Now may the God of patience and comfort grant you to be like-minded toward one an-other, according to Christ Jesus," Romans 15:5.

"Hatred stirs up strife, but love covers all sins," Proverbs 10:12.

"This is My commandment, that you love one another as I have loved you," John 15:12.

"But the fruit of the Spirit is love, joy, peace, longsuffering, kindness, goodness, faithfulness, gentleness, self-control. . . . If we live in the Spirit, let us also walk in the Spirit. Let us not become conceited, provoking one another, en-vying one another," Galatians 5:22-26.

"Beloved, let us love one another, for love is of God; and everyone who loves is born of God and knows God. He who does not love does not know God, for God is love. In this the love of God was manifested toward us, that God sent His only begotten Son into the world, that we might live through Him. In this is love, not that

we loved God, but that He loved us and sent His Son to be the propitiation for our sins. Beloved, if God so loved us, we also ought to love one another," 1 John 4:7-11.

"Love has been perfected among us in this: that we may have boldness in the day of judgment; because as He is, so are we in this world. There is no fear in love; but perfect love casts out fear, because fear involves torment," 1 John 4:17-18.

"Love suffers long and is kind; love does not envy; love does not parade itself, is not puffed up; does not behave rudely, does not seek its own, is not provoked, thinks no evil; does not rejoice in iniquity, but rejoices in truth; bears all things, believes all things, hopes all things, endures all things. Love never fails," 1 Corinthians 13:4-8.

STUDY GUIDE QUESTIONS

These questions are intended to help you gain insight and to further develop your battle plan. You might have to dig deep and face some frightening truths to answer them, but doing so will help you in the long run. I suggest reading the book in its entirety and then going through the questions, reading the corresponding chapter again if necessary. Recording your answers is also an excellent idea so you can refer back to them when the need arises. Be honest, be strong, and be vigilant in your prayers. Keep in mind that the devil using food against you and your loved ones is a long and drawn out war. It will not be easy and it will not be over after you have won a few battles. It could take months, years, or even a lifetime. Your goal is to gain more victories than defeats. You are now aware of the enemy and what he is doing, so you have finally leveled the playing field. Align yourself with God and you will gain the upper hand. In Jesus you have a strong and faithful ally who will help you ward off the enemy's attacks and lead you to victory.

Chapter 1 They Don't Call it Devil's Food for Nothing

1) Who have you been falsely accusing of contributing to your food issues? Identify where you place blame and release them from condemnation. Dig deep and be honest, as you may be subconsciously blaming loved ones for your diet dilemma.

2) Can you identify with Eve and her choice? Why do you think she opted to listen to Satan? Why do you?

3) Can you see similarities between Satan's tempting of Jesus and how he tempts you?

4) Will being aware of Satan's temptations help you resist? If so, why?

5) In what ways do food and drink have the potential to destroy us?

6) Given Daniel's blessing for resisting to partake in tainted offerings, can you see why it would be worth your while to avoid unhealthy foods? How might God bless you for resisting?

Chapter 2 Hell's in Your Kitchen

1) Over the course of your lifetime, how much time have you spent on discussions, thoughts, plans, and attempts to lose weight or alter your diet? What better things could you spend your time on that would bring you more joy, success, and productivity?

2) In what ways has the devil been keeping you from your purpose?

3) Have you been under the false assumption that you are immune to Satan's attacks? Can you now see ways that the enemy has been trying to hold you back physically and spiritually?

4) Have you given your food issues over to God? If not, why not? If so, what was your experience?

5) Have you ever thought the root cause of your eating habits could be the devil? How will having this information change your plan of action?

6) Take a peek in your kitchen. What evidence do you see of the enemy's presence?

7) Where does the devil hang around to tempt you on a regular basis? Can you think of all the places he visits, even infrequently, to coerce you into eating unhealthy?

8) Do your church-affiliated gatherings typically involve food? Is the food offered healthy and nourishing, a blessing from God, or is it meant to defile you from the inside out?

Chapter 3 Satan's Food Chain

1) What food items does Satan most often tempt you with?

- a) Write down common foods. **(My example is chocolate)**.

- b) Now list the descriptive ways he tempts you. **(Creamy, dark, sweet, hints of flavors, gooey, melting, rich).**

- c) Finally, write down what the foods actually consist of. **(Higher quality chocolate: Cocoa, sugar, vanilla bean. Lesser quality chocolate: sugar, chocolate, cocoa butter, milk fat, lactose, PGPR, vanillin, milk, artificial flavor, cocoa processed with alkali, and soy lecithin just to name a few).** Forcing yourself to look at what these seductive foods are actually made out of will break them down and remove the glamour, leaving you less susceptible to the hype.

2) Have you fallen for Satan's lie that you deserve junk food? Can you now see the truth? Write down why you do **not** deserve junk and why junk does **not** deserve you.

3) Are you a believer in the "just a little bit" lie? Balance and moderation are very important and it is vital that you eat foods you enjoy in a reasonable amount. Think of ways you can enjoy your favorites while not falling for the lie over and over again. **(I purchase a quality chocolate bar and have only 1-2 ounces, or squares, a day).**

4) Who truthfully knows about your struggles with food? Who are you hurting with your unhealthy eating habits?

5) Have you ever thought about Jesus facing temptation so He would be able to help you? Think about it now and decide what that means for you.

6) Write down reasons why what you eat does, in fact, matter. Why should you no longer delay making healthy choices?

7) Have you fallen for the lie that food is your comfort or that you're an emotional eater?

　　a) Why do you think it is so easy for you to believe?

　　b) How do you honestly feel after over-indulging? Do you truthfully feel the least bit comforted after the binge? Has food ever actually helped to solve a problem?

8) Are you using life's difficulties to justify your poor eating habits? If so, how is it damaging you? What can you do to get through the challenges of daily living that would be far more beneficial than eating junk food? Some ideas include praying, talking to family and friends, listening to music, writing in a journal, or going for a walk.

9) How often do you find yourself obsessing over food? How do you typically try to deal with it? Are your methods of distraction helpful or harmful? Can you see how obsessing

over food and weight actually inhibits your time and focus on the Lord?

10) Have you ever felt desperate for food? Admit and come to terms with some of the most embarrassing things you have done out of desperation. Can you see how the enemy, who is nothing more than a ruthless bully, would derive satisfaction from seeing you reduced to such levels over food? How would you benefit if you sank to your knees in prayer and turned immediately to God in those moments of desperation?

11) Why do you think gluttony is so over-looked in today's society? What can you do to combat it?

12) Do you feel guilty when you over eat? Most likely you have experienced both godly and worldly sorrow. Identify and write down the different feelings you have and where they come from; godly sorrow which can serve to help you, or worldly sorrow which harms you and keeps you down.

13) How can accepting your flaws and minor food slip ups actually help you move forward? Refer to 2 Corinthians 7:11.

14) Without any self-loathing, self-pitying, or getting defensive, can you see how carrying around extra weight negatively impacts your quality of life? Can you see that losing weight is not meant to change who you are, but rather how you are?

15) In what ways do you see your quality of life changing if you stop listening to the devil and his food lies?

16) Have you been under the misconception that you can control your eating habits? How has that actually hindered your success?

Chapter 4 Banishing the Enemy from Your Temple

1) Have you ever thought of your body as God's physical temple? Are there ways that you are desecrating His temple? What can you do to take good care of your body, His temple?

2) Are you destroying, with your food, the one for whom Christ died?

3) What changes can you make so that you are eating in a way that glorifies God?

4) How can you clean and polish your temple to get it into top shape, not for vanity's sake, but to glorify the Father?

5) Break bread with someone. Literally. Record how it makes you feel, both internally and toward the other person or people.

Chapter 5 In Defense of Chocolate

1) What food items do you thoroughly enjoy and hate the idea of giving up? Can you find healthier ways to consume these treats? A little research will go a long way.

2) Do you understand why spending money on quality ingredients rather than quantity of food can have a huge impact on your health? If you're not certain, pray about it and investigate on your own.

3) Make a conscious effort to sit down and truly savor a food that you typically enjoy. Eat it slowly.

4) Think about the different qualities of the food, such as taste and texture. Write down your thoughts, feelings, and observations before, during and after consuming it.

If you're not convinced, do your own experiment. Eat your favorite treat as you normally would. For many people that means eating quickly, efficiently, and mindlessly. Take note of how much you eat and how you feel after.

Compare those notes with your experience of savoring a treat, as described above.

Chapter 6 Going to Battle

1) When you think of waging war with the devil, what are your fears and concerns? List them and pray over each one.

2) How can you be certain that God will be victorious over the enemy? Take the time to seek out and write down scripture verses that convince you.

3) Are you ready to make the choice to ask Jesus for His help in the culinary battle? If you are ready to commit, let Him know.

4) Work on your food awareness. Be mindful of what you eat, where you eat, when you eat, and how much you eat. Pay attention to all of the food advertisements you see. It's a good idea to take some form of notes.

5) What emotions do you attach to food? Happiness? Sadness? Why do you believe that you associate these feelings with food? Food is an inanimate object. It is not capable of conjuring up any emotions or solving any problems. What you eat is meant to fuel your body

and that is all. Any thoughts or feelings you associate with food have been created by you or influences you have allowed.

6) Have you tried diets, supplements, or exercises recommended by others? How successful were your attempts?

7) Have you tried to ask for God's help with your food battles? If not, why? List reasons you have not given your culinary issues over to God. When you're finished, look them over. Do any of your reasons justify God not offering you help? Would anything justify God not coming to your aide? Hint, the answer is no!

8) Record your successes for praise and continued motivation. Record losses also, but only to learn from and not repeat them.

Chapter 7 Fighting for Others

1) Do you know of any friends or family members that are entrenched in the spiritual food battle? Have you prayed for them? If not, will you?

2) Have you exhibited poor eating habits in front of others? What are some things you can do to change those habits in order to set a better example?

3) If you have tried to set healthier eating examples, what kinds of opposition have you faced? If you have not yet attempted to make a change, be certain that you will face opposition. Where do you think such negativity stems from?

4) Why do you think it is so important for us to help others with love and compassion? The following questions are geared towards parents or those concerned with the health of children.

5) Is your child at a healthy, ideal weight? If you are not sure, please ask a physician.

176

Find out what a healthy weight range is for your child.

6) If your child is not at a healthy weight, it is time to be strong and fight for the health of your child. Start by forcing yourself to learn all of the diseases and medical problems your child is at a higher risk for. This should serve as a harsh wake up call to you. It is not meant to scare you, but rather to spur you into action. Know that you can reduce these risks and avoid possible problems for your child by doing something about it now.

7) What have you been doing, feeding, or allowing that has contributed to the excess weight your child carries? Be honest, the truth will allow you to be successful. Pray for God to open your eyes and reveal to you ways that you have been inadvertently harming your child's health.

8) What changes can you make to get your family on a healthier path? Ask for God's wisdom and strength to help you through these battles.

ABOUT THE AUTHOR

Nicole Grant has made her writing debut with *Feeding Demons*. She earned her Bachelor's degree in Psychology and shortly after took a detour into the world of physical fitness and well-being. Throughout years of working with a variety of clients, Nicole has witnessed the mental, physical, and spiritual battles that we are all faced with at one point or another. Every step of her journey has led to the creation of *Feeding Demons*. Nicole is excited to finally have found the courage to follow her passion of writing. She is dedicated to being the best wife, mom, and student and servant of Christ that she can be; and as we all know, some days are better than others!

For more insight and help with your battle, please visit the website: www.feedingdemonsbook.com.

88718552R00105

Made in the USA
Lexington, KY
16 May 2018